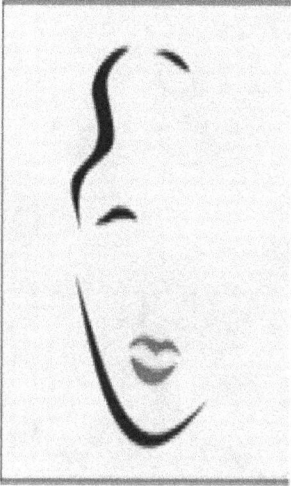

# You're Not Crazy!
## It's Menopause

**Marcia Williams**

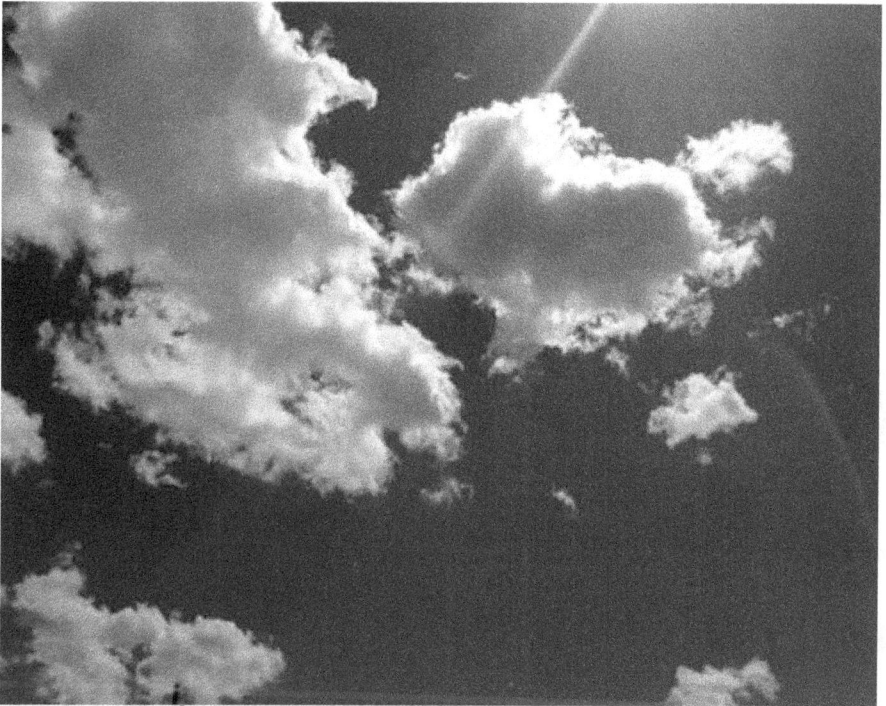

Forward by Sylvia Gates-Carlisle, MD

As I approached by fiftieth birthday, I gravitated toward certain kinds of women: positive, life affirming, evolving. When my kids lived at home, involvement in their activities opened my world to their friends' parents. I now had the opportunity to re-evaluate who I wanted in my life.

I met Marcia by accident and found her a blessing. We could talk about our lives authentically and support each other. The folks in my life who wanted to complain and criticize, I needed to walk away from. In the face of life's challenges, they were blind to blessings. Their negativity was contagious, as the Bible teaches: "Do not be deceived: Bad company ruins good morals." (*1 Corinthians 15:33ESV*).

Each day is a new opportunity to learn and thrive, or shrivel and whine. Join Marcia on the "Second Spring" journey.

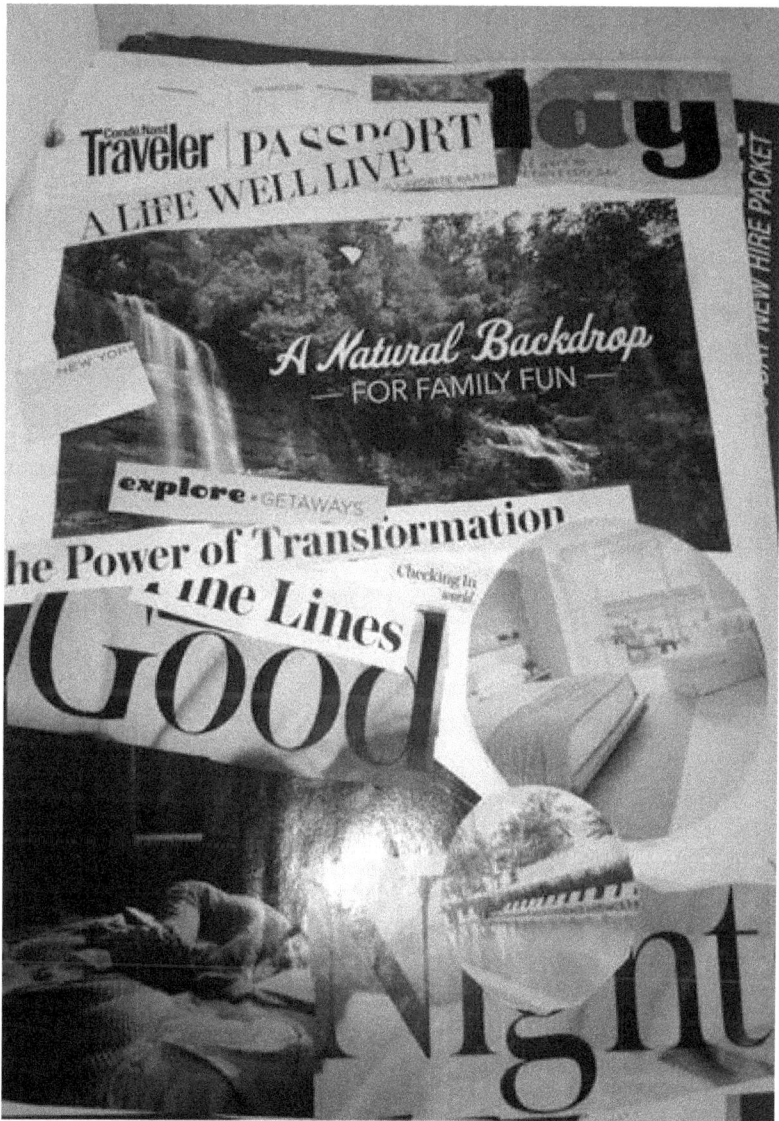

This is my vision board; you might create your own vision board to see where you would like to be in your life and whether or not you are close to achieving this goal.

## Important

The material in this book is for informational purposes only and is not recommended to diagnose or treat menopause. Please consult your health provider in all matters concerning menopausal symptoms. Neither the publisher nor the author directly or indirectly dispenses medical advice, nor do we prescribe any remedies or assume any responsibility for those who choose to treat themselves.

# Dedication, and Acknowledgments

This book is dedicated:

To my husband, Al Williams, who went on this journey with me. Though at times challenging, you never faltered in your love for me, and I thank you always for being there.

To my adult children, Nicole, Shaun and my son-In-Law Tobias, whose patience and tolerance gave me the encouragement to complete this book. I was able to write so that other children can understand how to deal with their mothers in a loving and respectful way, while their mothers are traveling through their menopausal journey.

To my lovely grandchildren, Atlas and Ayleigh, from whom I have learned that love is unconditional. Your smiles and energy fuel me and keep me moving forward, so that I can enjoy you with happiness and balance.

To my friend, Sylvia Gates-Carlisle, M.D., who has been there since the beginning of our "Second Spring" journey when we vowed not to let menopause get the best of us.

And to my sister-in-law, Sherry Smith-Williams, oh my goodness! I thank you so much for your knowledge and editing expertise. Without you I couldn't have seen the vision of my book come alive, and I appreciate all your effort and time.


You're Not Crazy! It's Menopause

# Table of Contents

# *Introduction:* Growing Up in the Hood

My name is Marcia Williams, and I've been a cosmetologist for over twenty years. The reason I became a cosmetologist is that I wanted to be a business owner. While visiting a childhood friend at her salon in San Francisco, I spent the whole day observing her and her business. She was self-employed, making good money and keeping her own schedule. After observing her, I went back home and signed up at Sacramento City College for Cosmetology. And that's initially why I wanted to be a cosmetologist; I saw it as lucrative and as a way to become a business owner.

However, when I actually began working in this profession, I found that it allowed me to establish unique and intimate relationships with the women who sought my services. I have developed personal relationships with my clients, because they know that they can trust me, no matter what they want to talk about. It was very important to me to give them the assurance that we could TALK, without their being judged by me.

So I found myself listening to a wide range of stories, problems, situations, and so on. At first, when I listened and heard what these women were going through, I would say to myself, "My life is not so bad!" I later understood that just by thinking that way I was judging. I prayed not to do that but rather to listen with my whole heart, and when I did I was able to show concern and keep an open mind. Now I am slow to speak and fast to listen, and this has helped me in my own life as well.

### *From the Stylist's Chair*

As a cosmetologist, I speak with a lot of women in and out of the salon. I have found that a lot of women are taking medications prescribed to them by their doctors, while not fully taking care of the issue at hand: menopause. For instance, one day a young lady thirty-three years of age, whom I had not seen for a long while, walked into the salon. I

1

asked her where she had been. She said "I was in the hospital for a hysterectomy, and after being released, I took a whole bottle of prescription Tylenol tablets." My response was "Oh no, why?" And she said, "I was tired of being tired."

I asked her what she meant. She said she didn't know! And yet: after two more days in the hospital, she had been released, this time with a prescription for sleeping pills and another for Ambutol. It was incredible to me that she had been sent home with that type of medication when she had just tried to commit suicide. I asked her if she had had any counseling after her hysterectomy. She seemed to have gone right into artificial menopause, a symptom of which is depression. She said they had just sent her home with medication.

On another occasion, one of my clients came into the salon, running late and furious! I said "Mary, calm down." I asked, "What's wrong with you?" The reason I was so surprised is that Mary was usually a kind and happy person when she came to the salon. She exclaimed, "I just about ran this person off the road, they were driving so slow in front of me! I was trying to get to my hair appointment on time!" I said "What? You're kidding, right? You know that's road rage!" Now Mary was in her late forties.

She said, "No, and I forgot to take my antidepressant this morning! I have no patience anymore; I don't know what's up with me." Well, I asked her if she had had her hormone levels checked, and she responded, "I never thought of that!" I asked, because impatience is another symptom of menopause.

I remembered after my mother had her hysterectomy, things were not the same after that. I noticed that my mom wasn't her usual self. She started to yell a lot, and at times I saw her in another light: not as happy, for some reason or another. I am not saying my mom had always been happy, but for the most part she had been a very strong and positive person. Something was different. I knew she went through a lot, but I never saw her sweat about it. Now for some reason it was starting to show; the anxiety of life was starting to take a toll on her.

2

If these women (including my mom in her time) had had counseling to educate them on menopausal symptoms and the options of hormone replacement, herbs or medication, at least they would have had choices. They would have had an explanation for their behaviors and would have understood themselves better. Instead they were in the dark, playing a guessing game as to what was going on.

## Bringing it Home

I grew up in a housing project named Hunter's Point in San Francisco during the late 60s and early 70s. My mother, Goldie Toups, a single mother of four children, was an awesome woman. What was so amazing about her was that she did this—raising four children alone—with a smile. And she could make me laugh so hard that tears would come down my face. She shared her experiences of everyday life with humor and wit.

We later moved to the housing project of Sunnydale. The move was a good change for our family, because Sunnydale had beautiful— clean buildings, green grass—and it was walking distance from our school. The housing project used to be for men in the military and their families, so the government had maintained the facility well until they turned it over to the City.

Over time, however, crack cocaine found its way into the neighborhood; murders and robberies started to take place; and the neighborhood became a rough and violent environment. Yet, despite this, I remember having a great childhood. I had plenty of friends and never needed or wanted for much. I don't know how, but my mother provided for us physically, mentally, and lovingly, always with a smile on her face. Her deep faith may have contributed to her strength in providing for the family.

My mother was a bus driver for San Francisco Municipal during a time when the majority of drivers were men, and routes were dangerous (especially during the night shifts). She did what she had to do to take care of her family, something I have always thought took unbelievable courage. She taught me to have thick skin, because you have to go through some tough times in your life.

In her later days, however, my mother began to encounter illness. She had been so busy caring for us that, by the time she was diagnosed with diabetes, she was so ill as to need daily insulin shots. In her late 40s, she underwent a hysterectomy, which likely precipitated an artificial menopause, and, from that time on, I observed that her manner began to change. A woman with a heart of gold, who never complained about anything, now suddenly became irritable—and would yell at whoever would listen (or not)—and curse at the drop of a hat.

I was not sure how to deal with my mother's sometimes hot, sometimes cold personality. She was, at certain times, mean; she was a lot more serious about life; and the laughter was becoming less and less frequent. I now understand she was experiencing mood swings. Though my mother and I talked about everything under the sun, she never mentioned menopause. Her silence leads me to believe, she didn't know what was happening to her.

In the 1970s many women frequently did not receive education about hormone imbalances or about how to take care of themselves during menopause. They had limited access to health care. The mothers of my friends acted similarly, most of them also marginalized single mothers. Some had a more difficult time than others, but if we kids had only known what was up and why our mothers acted the way they did, it would have been so much better.

I had a friend whose mother once had a great shape and a keen sense of fashion. She cooked a fantastic spaghetti, which I later learned was enhanced with sugar and ketchup to make it taste good for the kids! But all of a sudden she was huge; I mean, it seemed to happen overnight. I asked my friend, "What's going on with your mom?" She said that her mother was taking some medicine that made her that way. She didn't know what the medicine was for, but it seemed to calm her down.

I had never known her mother to act out in any way, but for a period my friend had gone to live with her grandparents while her

4

mother was in the hospital for a mental evaluation. When her mother returned home a couple of months later, she was taking medication, and that was when she started gaining weight. Her behavior finally became so out of control that my friend's grandparents had to have her committed.

Could this have been that she had a hormonal imbalance but was mistakenly diagnosed and prescribed medication, such as an antidepressant, for mental illness? In any case, she finally had to live the rest of her life with the stigma of mental health issues.

After becoming a cosmetologist, I heard many stories about women who had "symptoms but no solutions." I decided to do some research, and I asked questions of the professionals. I wanted to discover, for myself, how a woman can live a sane life of balance and wellness.

I am writing this book for women who are experiencing or who will experience menopause. I wish to educate those who seek to understand "the guest" that will be arriving in their lives. This guest is coming; one just doesn't know when.

We need to come together and let our womenfolk know about this life intrusion. They need to equip themselves with the tools to handle "the change," so that they can share this awareness with family members who may not know what is happening. My goal is to educate women on how they can sail through this period of life--this journey— easily and happily.

### Knowledge is Power

**Premature (Early) Menopause** means the unexpected early onset of menopause. A woman typically experiences the symptoms of peri-menopause before the age of forty-five.

**Peri-Menopause** means the time prior to menopause when hormonal changes are occurring and our menstrual periods become irregular.

5

Onset may be accompanied by cholesterol changes, sleep changes, hot flashes, and bone loss. When these symptoms occur, it is advisable to get other tests—such as thyroid, pregnancy, and so on—to rule out other causes. Please consult your OB-GYN or doctor.

**Artificial Menopause** means the termination of menstrual periods by other than natural means: radiation, surgery or other procedure.

**Menopause** means the cessation of menstrual cycles. Peri-menopause symptoms can last up to three years and continue even after menstrual periods stop.

**Post-Menopause** means the years after the cessation of menstrual cycles.

Ladies, if you are experiencing symptoms, please see your OB-GYN or doctor to get your hormone levels checked. Though your hormonal levels may still change, at least you will know where to start and what to do.

In my case, I went to a compound pharmacy in Sacramento and talked with the pharmacist there. I asked for information regarding BHRT (Bio-identical Hormone Replacement Therapy). Once I gained the knowledge, I went to my OB-GYN and discussed what I was going through. I told her that, after talking with the pharmacist, I thought I would like a prescription for hormone replacement therapy (low estrogen, higher doses of progesterone and some testosterone). So I went to my doctor with a solution to my situation and removed all the guess work; remember doctors only spend about 15 minutes with you.

When you go to your doctor with a plan, it makes it easier for them to help you resolve your problem. Educate yourselves about your body needs before you go to the doctor instead of relying on them. I know it's sad to say, because you go to the doctor for an expert opinion. However, nowadays you have to be your own advocate.

With knowledge and the implementation of a healthy lifestyle, we can bring ourselves back to the whole person we once were. Knowing just how menopause changed my mother's life, I was able to equip myself with the tools needed to refuse to succumb to this intrusion without a fight.

In the following pages, I will introduce you to the nature of menopause and offer you a number of tools for dealing with it. I will sketch out a road map to a sane life of balance and wellness. We will cover hormone replacement therapy, diet, natural remedies, high fashion and fabulous hair styles, along with the social and spiritual aspects of living the best life possible. Each chapter will focus on one tool, with stories "from the stylist's chair," a little insight from my own life, and the knowledge that will empower you to make positive adjustments in your own life.

### What the Experts Say

According to the North American Menopause Society, by the year 2000, 45.6 million American women will have reached menopause age, and the number is expected to increase every year to 1.1 billion women by year 2025. Joan Borysenko, Ph.D., says that during this stage of life women are most likely to seek peace of mind against a tense background of turmoil and change. It is a period during which they may have affairs, end twenty plus years of marriage, get left by partners, face empty nest syndrome, discover new aspects of their identity, and so on. They are also less likely to make excuses for others and more apt to tell the truth.

As women, we experience and deal with things differently. It is important that once we experience unusual personality or behavioral changes, we investigate ourselves—body, mind and soul—to see what is happening and determine how to make the necessary adjustments.

### What Do You Think?

1. How do you feel about your journey with menopause?
2. What actions have you taken to make this a positive journey?

3. What physical and mental changes do you feel that you have been through since the beginning of this journey?

As you work through this book, I will provide you with questions that will allow you to begin a journey of self-investigation and life change. It will be up to you to do the work, whatever it takes, but I believe you will find that your well-being is worth it.

Now that I have experienced menopause, I have so much empathy for my mother and what she went through. What great endurance she had and displayed in her lifetime, without the benefit of hormonal replacement therapy and other essential tools for coping with menopause! It is a strength that I have been able to pass on to my daughter and, in turn, she will pass on to hers.

Thank you, Mom, for the strength and courage that you bequeathed me.

Love you, Mom!

# Chapter 1 You are Worth It!

When I embarked on the journey of menopause, I remember feeling irritable, sweaty and depressed for what seemed like no reason at all. It is a serious situation when you find yourself asking, "What is my life worth here? What is my purpose?" Or when you are too tired even to worry about it, too tired to go on with life as usual.

Recognizing the onset of menopause, I decided to find out what could help me on this journey. As it is for many women, menopause can be a difficult journey, but it need not end badly.

## From the Stylist's Chair

One of my clients, Lori, had been on antidepressants for many years because of an incident that had happened to her while she attended college. Now, she was getting older and weight gain from taking the medication was becoming obvious. What were the doctors going to give her now?

I remember her telling me a story about how one night she woke up in the middle of the night and could not sleep. She was saying that her husband was going to leave her, because she could not have children. They had been married for years, and now he was bringing this up. I asked her why it was an issue now.

Lori was in her late forties and going through menopause. The onset of menopause seemed to have exacerbated her other problems and was making life more difficult for her. Although her husband had accepted the fact that they could not have kids a long time ago, this had now become an issue for him, out of the blue.

Depression was at an all-time high, and she continually reflected back on the past. When she went to her doctor with the story, she told me, her doctor increased the dosage of her medications. I asked her if she had seen her OB-GYN, and she said, "No." I suggested she see her

OB-GYN to get her hormone levels checked and obtain some type of hormone replacement therapy. Even if one has been diagnosed with severe depression from other causes, menopause can add to it.

So Lori went to her OB-GYN and asked her about menopause symptoms and if hormone replacement therapy might help her. She asked if the doctor could prescribe her such a course of treatment to help her reduce some of her depression, and the doctor did. With that said, Lori wasn't a hundred percent, but she was acting and feeling better. She joined Weight Watchers and started losing weight. So at least she was concentrating on bettering herself and not focused solely on her past, making it a bigger issue than it was. The right diagnosis can help you handle life in a more positive way.

### Bringing It Home

When I first started experiencing the symptoms of depression, I had been married for over 20 years. Though my husband is a good husband and would tell me and show me that he loved me, it seemed not to matter. I started telling him that he did not love me, and then I would cry uncontrollably for hours, trying to figure out why. He would tell me, "Honey, I love you no matter what you're going through."

At this time in my life I didn't know what was going on. I had been a happy and cheerful person—ask anyone! So, I went to the doctor and explained what I was going through. I also felt depressed, unattractive, and my self-confidence was abandoning me as fast as menopause was coming on. The doctor told me I was going through depression—like a midlife crisis. She prescribed Wellbutin, Xanax and Valium.

I can remember clearly that when I was discussing what was going on in my life, she told me, "Oh, you just need something to take the edge off, something for anxiety." Believe me, she had no problem prescribing these medications. When I started reading the side effects, I said to myself that by the time I am finished with these medicines, I would surely be sick, tried and confused even more. These side effects were going to add to the grief I was already going through.

10

As an example of these side effects, clearly stated on the bottle, printed as big as day: "WARNING: this medication may cause seizures, high blood pressure, heart palpitations..." and so on. When I did start taking the medicine, I felt worst. I didn't want to do anything but sleep my life away.

So I got tired of that and started researching what was going on with these high emotions. After describing these symptoms to a client who is an OB-GYN specializing in Bio-identical Hormone Replacement Therapy (BHRT), I discovered I was going through peri-menopause. It was then that I did some research and went to my OB-GYN to request hormone replacement therapy. I kid you not: Afterwards, I felt eighty percent better and was getting a good night's sleep.

In this way, I began my "marathon for menopause," researching to find out what this thing called menopause was and why it was affecting me and my family so drastically. I knew nothing about this rite of passage, when, at age 46, I encountered it, this transitional journey that one embarks on in a moment's notice, sending your hormones into flux.

I found myself experiencing a major change in life, a change quite unfamiliar to me. I embarked on new, unexplored territory with weight gain, hot flashes, moodiness, loss of hormones, which —taken together—made me unpleasant to be around. Then it hit me; I was experiencing what my mother and countless other women before me had experienced: the unknown and unwanted guest of menopause.

I refused to accept menopause as a stage in life for which there was no successful treatment. There had to be something to treat women going through this experience to make our lives more enjoyable. I started reading books and asking other women what their experiences were. Those who had experienced menopause all seemed to have the symptoms but no answers.

Most of them went to their doctors and explained what was going on in their lives and were prescribed medication such as an antidepressant. A lot of women I talked to were misdiagnosed with depression when what they needed was to get their hormone levels checked.

I was already wary of taking medicines prescribed with little consideration of the conditions for which they were prescribed and their possible side-effects. I had had an earlier bout with high blood pressure and experienced actually passing out when I took the medication prescribed for me. Luckily my husband, Al, was with me. He was able to take me to the car, and I laid down until I felt better.

After that, I vowed to do whatever it took to get my blood pressure down, and I soon no longer took high blood pressure medicine. Although I had a family history of high blood pressure, I decided not to be a statistic. By educating myself and making changes in my life, I overcame the ailment to which I was genetically prone. It was my goal to show that the cycle could be broken.

So when menopause hit and I was prescribed an antidepressant, I made the decision to stop taking the pills prescribed for me, which made me feel worse than I had felt prior to the diagnosis. While taking the pills, I felt like a lifeless woman.

I was determined to find a way to go through this "Second Spring" of life—menopause—feeling great and looking good! As a cosmetologist, I had the opportunity to ask different women about their experiences with menopause. Some did not even know they were going through it; some did not want to know. I found that some women talk about it, and some do not. Well, I want to talk about it.

Menopause just appeared in my life. I was doing well in life and all of the sudden, here comes weight gain, moodiness, hot flashes, excessive menstruation, fibroids—oh my goodness!—the list goes on. How could I see myself as a beautiful woman, as a beautiful human being, when all of this was going on?

I had to get to the bottom of it, because I knew it was not normal; there was nothing about this that was sane. I wanted to find out what it takes to enjoy life while still going through this menopausal part of life. From the stories women told me, I began to realize that balance is the key to stability. That's why it is always good to check in on yourself to see how you are doing.

Ask yourself: Am I as nice to others as I could be? Do others enjoy being around me? Do I smile to make others feel happy, in turn bringing joy to myself? There are hundreds of questions you can ask yourself, or others, in order to do a check in.

If you discover you are encountering menopause, then you can do whatever it takes to get better and feel good. It can be done, and you are worth it.

Let's not be afraid of this condition; it is a part of womanhood. We need to put menopause in its place. If menopause is embraced and handled right, we can achieve a healthy attitude and adopt beneficial practices even during this difficult stage of our life.

You too can be a more loveable, pleasant woman going through the change. You needn't find yourself scared of aging, because this process actually is one of the best parts of life —a woman's experience of menopause can be, in fact, a thing of real beauty.

### Knowledge is Power

As always, check with your doctor. Go to the doctor with a potential solution, so that you and the doctor can discuss together what will help to alleviate what you're going through. In addition, there are workshops and seminars on these subjects, where you might listen to professionals and others experiencing the same kinds of things.

Because you will be around other women that are going through similar situations, you can bounce ideas and stories off one another, and you will realize that you are not alone. Getting out may help to bring you back to sanity.

Other interventions you might try include: herbs, compound creams, vitamins and magnesium and/or zinc. But always consult your doctor before taking these.

According to the *New World Dictionary of the American Language*, "menopause" means: the permanent cessation of menstruation, normally between the ages of 40 and 50, or the period during which this occurs; female climacteric, or change of life.

Normally you will experience menopause after the age of 35, be it natural or artificial (brought on by a full or partial hysterectomy). However, now we know that women can experience menopause at any age....

**Listed here—but not limited to these— are some symptoms of menopause:**

Body aches and pains
Lack of concentration
Short memory lapses
Weight gain
Loss of muscle tone
Problems with urination
Fatigue
Dizziness
Changes in skin
Anxiety
Nervousness
Changes in emotions
Depression
Irritability
Moody
Loss in sex drive
Painful intercourse
Dryness in vagina
Hot flashes
Sleep problems
Night sweats
Weird dreams
Vaginal odor
Flatulence

Indigestion
Aching ankles, knees and shoulders
Sore heals
Snoring
Vertigo
Skin feeling crawly
Thinning scalp*

Wow, look at what we're dealing with! And we have to look good on top of all this! No wonder we are STRONG, AND INVINCIBLE!!!!!!!!!!!!!!!!!

* I am indebted to Althea J. Jackson, M.D., for this list of menopausal symptoms.

**What the Experts Say**

This is what the experts say about using antidepressants: "WARNING: Antidepressants may increase the risk of suicidal thoughts or actions in women. However, depression and certain other mental problems may also increase the risk of suicide. Talk with the patient's doctor to be sure that the benefits outweigh the risks." OMG!!!!!!

There are about 454 million women in the United States taking antidepressants. If you have concerns about side effects, call your doctor for medical advice.

To have your hormone levels checked, consult your OB-GYN. For information about BRHT, check with a compound pharmacist; they are the experts in the field ....

While the research is still out on the ultimate cause of menopause, what is known is that by our late forties and early fifties our estrogen levels drop about 50%; progesterone levels drop about 75%; and testosterone 50%. There is also a sharp decline in melatonin; this hormone chemically causes drowsiness and lowers the body temperature, which helps us get a good night's sleep. These hormonal changes in our bodies are typically accompanied by the symptoms of peri-menopause.

### What Do You Think?

1. Have you ever felt depressed for a reason you could not identify?

2. Have you ever experienced changes in other people that you could not explain?

3. Do you know the symptoms of menopause? Do you know what to look for?

4. Do you have a plan for dealing with these symptoms?

5. Do you have a role model for how to manage menopause whose example you can draw from?

6. If you are experiencing three or more symptoms of menopause, can you focus on eliminating one at a time?

7. Are you willing to approach your doctor with some solutions you learned of that may help you during your peri-, post-, or menopausal journey?

8. How will you approach your health care provider? (humble, heartfelt, and with deep concerns about your well-being?)

### Further Reading

Collins, Joseph. *What's Your Menopause Type?* Roseville, California: Prima Health, 2000.

Love, Susan. *Menopause and Hormone Book: Making Informed Choices*. New York, New York: Random House, 1997.

Northrup, Christiane. *Women's Bodies, Women's Wisdom: Creating Physical and Emotional Health and Healing*. New York, New York: Bantam Books, 2010.

Rosenthal, M. Sara. *Natural Woman's Guide to Hormone Replacement Therapy: An Alternative Approach*.Franklin Lakes, New Jersey: New Page Books, 2003.

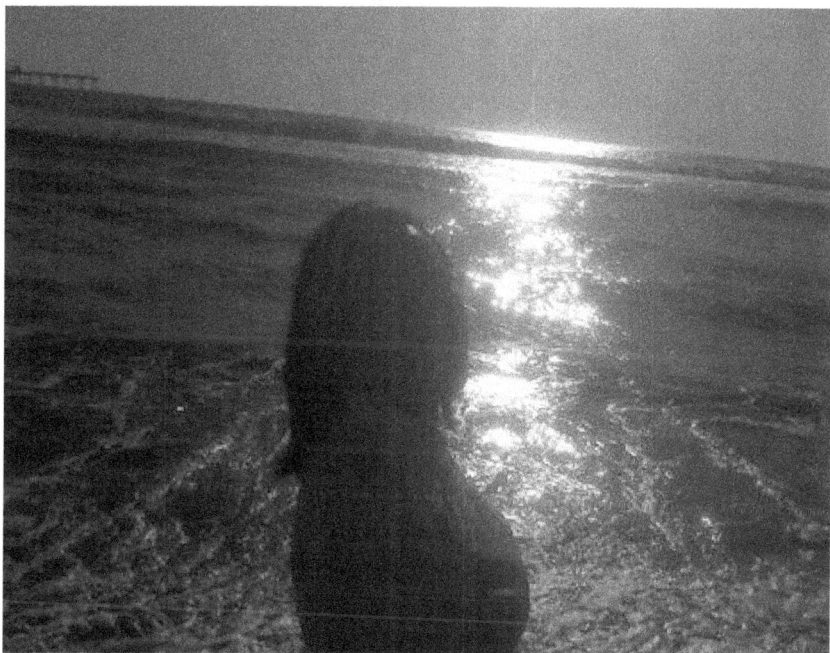

# Chapter 2 A Sane Life of Balance and Wellness

When I realized that I was going through peri-menopause, I decided, for myself, to do some research and ask some questions of health professionals. I wanted to discover how I could live a sane life of balance and wellness. To start with, I learned that our bodies are made up of all different sorts of hormones, and these hormones often become imbalanced in menopause. My hormones were out of control, wacko!

### From the Stylist's Chair

I can remember talking to Bernice, one of my clients, some time ago. I went to her home to interview her about menopause, and, at that point in my research, I just wanted to know how other women were handling the journey. Bernice is a Registered Nurse (RN), and she cares a lot about others. She stressed that she worried so much about others that her menopause situation had taken a back seat. It got so severe that she had to do something about it.

With the night sweats and the hot flashes, it was driving her crazy. She could not focus on what she loved doing. At the time, she owned her own daycare, because she also had a passion for children. She had her own business taking care of children when all the sudden it hit! Her menopause! Of course she knew it was coming, because she was experiencing fibroid issues and had surgery to remove them (although it didn't help because apparently they came right back).

I shared with her my experience of Bio-identical Hormone Replacement Therapy (BHRT) compound creams, and she decided to try them out. To her surprise, they helped significantly. She had approached her physician and explained to her what she wanted; she went to her physician with the facts about the hormones she needed, and, with that, the physician was able to give her an appropriate prescription.

One important note: When asking your OB-GYN for compound hormones, share your knowledge of the facts about BHRT. When you go to your specialist with facts and possible doses—which you can get from the results of your hormone level testing or from a compound pharmacist—your OB-GYN has something solid to work from. You might approach your pharmacist first with your symptoms, and the pharmacist can recommend or suggest how much is needed to start. That way you have something to go to your physician with.

Honestly, your physician may not be well-versed in this area. Instead of admitting this, he or she might be reluctant to prescribe BHRT. The pharmacist's recommendation will encourage your physician to pursue the possibility.

### Bringing It Home

I can remember when I first realized that something was out of balance with me. At the time, I had just opened my second salon and everything was going according to schedule. One day, for some reason, I was feeling all of Evilene ("evil"-ene), an aspect of my personality I had not experienced before peri-menopause.

I had hired several stylists, and a couple of them were not working out. They were not a good fit for an Image Salon. That day, one of them had started to act unprofessional. After she left, I just packed her stuff into a box.

When she showed up a couple of days later, like everything was all good, she walked passed me, where I was sitting at the reception desk. I asked her, "Where are you going?"

She responded, "I'm going to my station." I told her that she could no longer work for me and that she was fired! She said, "Whatever, I still need to get my stuff." I kicked the box I had packed earlier to her. I told her that there was no need; I had packed her stuff for her. Now, that was just mean on my part.

Too bad she had to experience that. I do not want Evilene to show her face in my life ever again. That was awful! I would apologize to that woman if I saw her again. However, I found out that she had since passed away from ovarian cancer. I had known she had it and was in remission. Maybe that's why she was acting inappropriately, with a "don't care" attitude.

As for me, I now know what my problem was. If I had been a kinder person at that time, I could have explored her feelings and worked it out. However, I thought that what I did was the best way to handle it. Fire with explosion! I was wrong, and I'm glad I can admit my mistakes and move on with my life to become a better person.

During the process of menopause and aging, we lose some of the hormones and enzymes that make up our bodies. We have to know how to replace them. The three main hormones involved in hormone replacement are estrogen, progesterone and testosterone. They can be replaced through hormone replacement therapy. Enzymes can be replaced by eating vegetables, especially raw vegetables (see Chapter 3).

My mother never had the benefit of hormone replacement therapy. After she underwent a hysterectomy, she had no consultation on what to expect or education regarding hormone levels in the body. She was sent home to heal with only pain pills. When I encountered menopause, I sought an alternative path and set about to break the cycle.

After some research, I went to my OB-GYN and asked her to prescribe a dose of each hormone in proportion to the normal level of hormones in the female hormonal system. We started with low doses to see how my body would react and gradually increased the doses, as needed. Two hormones were applied in cream form (estrogen and testosterone) and one was taken in pill form (progesterone). Hormone replacement creams were the best thing that happened to me after starting out on the menopausal journey....

### Knowledge is Power

Hormones are chemical substances that have a significant biological presence in both men and women. Hormones are produced and released by specific body tissues; these releases are in short bursts. There is no schedule for when hormones are released; they can be released at any minute or hour. The release of hormones can also happen during a menstrual cycle. Once released, the hormones travel through the body to other tissues, using the circulatory system, where they influence growth and behavior.

*Estrogen* is a female hormone produced in the ovaries, and it is the primary sex hormone of childbearing women. In essence, estrogen consists of a group of three hormones that are important for reproductive cycles (menstrual and estrous). These three estrogens occur naturally in women: estrone, estradiol, and estriol. They are present in the body during pre-pregnancy and from when the female first starts her menstrual cycle until menopause. Originally, estradiol is the predominant estrogen. During pregnancy, estriol becomes the predominant estrogen, and during post-menopause, estrone becomes predominant.

*Progesterone* is a female hormone that helps with libido and is instrumental in maintaining pregnancy. Progesterone is produced in the ovaries and the adrenal glands. It is also produced in the placenta when a woman is pregnant. This hormone is important for preparation of the lining of the uterus for pregnancy by causing the inner membrane of the uterus to generate special proteins to receive and nurture fertilized eggs. If no egg is received, menstruation will come. Progesterone helps to regulate the menstrual cycle.

*Testosterone* is a hormone that is produced in both men and women. In women, testosterone is produced in the ovaries and the adrenal glands. Although testosterone helps to facilitate the libido in both men and women, in women it also contributes to the sensitivity of their clitoris and nipples. Testosterone is important for promoting bone and muscle strength, healthy hair, and good energy levels as well. Since the ovaries help to produce testosterone, removal of the ovaries (through a hysterectomy) can result in a decrease in bone and muscle strength, and lower energy levels.

It is insightful to learn what your body is going through with hormonal imbalances. Hormones in your body are like gas in a car. Without the replacement of hormones, our bodies run sluggish or stop running entirely. You're exhausted, just tired, and don't know where to

21

start. You're wondering, "When will all of this end?" When your hormones are out of balance, it will show up in your behavior and attitude towards life.

By our late forties and early fifties, our estrogen levels drop dramatically, about 50%. There is so much going on in our lives during this time of midlife that going through menopause is often confused with issues caused by other factors. So we can eliminate some of the guess work by going to our doctors and/ or doing the research to find out what gives our bodies balance, whether it's hormone therapy, diet, or exercise.

Here are some of the benefits that one may get from hormone replacement: youthful skin, balanced moods (fewer emotional ups and downs, less irritability), less vaginal dryness, less anxiety, less depression, less confusion, less fogginess, more energy, more stamina, no more hot flashes, no more night sweats, better memory, somewhat normal sex drive, and much needed sleep!

At the same time, we need to get to know our own bodies and how they respond to different hormone therapies and other interventions. What works for one person, doesn't necessarily work for another. In my personal quest, hormone creams (which you get from a compound pharmacy as prescribed by a doctor) were critical. They kept me physically and mentally stable. Without these creams, I would have been a virtual monster--which is to put it mildly.

You can check with your doctor about having your hormone levels checked and to inquire what form of BHRT or what creams are right for you. You can also speak with a pharmacist who is a compound specialist.

Aside from the creams I used, I also kept a menopausal survival kit, which consisted of, but was not limited to: cotton face towels, dry pajamas or gowns (all made of 100% cotton), and a mineral spray mist for my face, just in case my body temperature got too hot! I kept these items in my nightstand, so I could be prepared for my night sweats. And also, I kept on hand a bottle of melatonin for sleepless nights, and a miniature fan. I called this my menopausal survival kit. Just being prepared helps!

Remember ladies, we are not just dealing with the estrogen hormone; we are dealing with the lost progesterone (which helps the distribution of estrogen), testosterone (which may help us think more logically), and a loss of libido.

**What the Experts Say**

According to Ellis Quinn Youngkin, much controversy about using hormone therapy has arisen from the Women's Health Initiative findings of 2002. This 15-year study of post-menopausal women found that women using BHRT showed a higher incidence of coronary heart disease, strokes, blood clots in the lung, and invasive breast cancer. These findings caused many women to be confused about or even scared to use hormone therapy.

In light of studies such as these, what is the current advice about using hormone therapy? Every woman is different, and any therapy should be geared to her individual health history, heredity and lifestyle needs. If used appropriately, hormone therapy can help with sleep disturbances, physical functioning, and body pain. Consult your OB-GYN or doctor to see if this option is good for you.

**What Do You Think?**

1. Should you explore the option of HRT creams?

2. Is this worth it for your family and yourself?

3. Will you look into more information about Bioidentical Hormone Replacement Therapy?

4. Can you ask more questions that will make you more comfortable while using BHRT?

23

5. Is there cancer in your family that may increase your chances of getting cancer due to taking estrogen for a short period of time?

6. Should you seek help from a naturopathic doctor that specializes in BHRT and its effects?

7. Can you research more on Bioidentical Hormone Replacement Therapy by looking on the internet?

8. Should you look into the idea of taking progesterone, estrogen and testosterone all at once in a cream to save yourself money rather than taking estrogen alone?


### Further Reading

Goldstein, Steven R. and Laurie Ashner. *Could It Be......Perimenopause? How Women 35-50 Can Overcome Forgetfulness, Mood Swings, Insomnia, Weight Gain, Sexual Dysfunction, and Other Telltale Signs of Hormonal Imbalance*. Boston, Massachusetts: Little Brown and Company, 1998, 2000.

Harpaz, Mickey. *Menopause Reset!* Emmaus, Pennsylvania: Rodale, 2011.

Perricone, Nicholas. *The Wrinkle Cure: Unlock the Power of Cosmeceuticals for Supple, Youthful Skin*. New York, New York: First Warner Books, 2001.

Posner, Trisha. *No Hormones, No Fear: A Natural Journey through Menopause*. New York, New York: Villard, 2002.

Wingert, Pat and Barbara Kantrowitz. *The Menopause Book*. New York, New York: Thomas Allen and Son Limited, 2006, 2009.

Youngkin, Ellis Quinn. *What about Using Hormone Therapy for Menopausal Symptoms?*

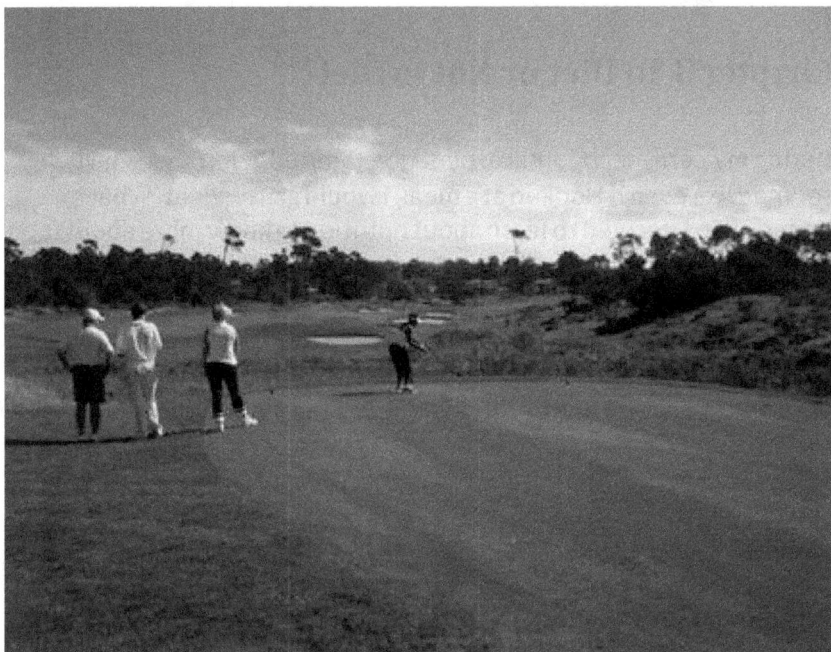

Golfing at Pebble Beach....this is sane and well balanced for me. I love playing golf.

# Chapter 3 To Diet or Not to Diet?

During my peri-menopausal experience, I started gaining weight. It seemed like even if I looked at a meal, I would gain weight. What a tragedy! So I decided to learn about nutrition to know more about food and how food could benefit me. This was a great idea, as not only did I learn what was beneficial to eat from a nutritional point of view but I also learned what foods are good for weight loss. Most successful weight loss is planned and takes preparation. The more you plan your meals—serving size and nutritional value—the more successful you will be.

### From the Stylist's Chair

Oh, what a fun time we had that day! It was the beginning of a healthy lifestyle for me. I met up with one of my clients and her friend, Denise, at Denise's house at 8:00 am on Thanksgiving Day. We planned to carpool to the "Race to Feed the Hungry," one of the biggest races in the United States. This was the first time I had run with some 25,000 people or more, here in Sacramento!

In the days before the race, I was anxious and wanted to prepare as much as possible. So I would drive down to the Capital Building in Sacramento; park; then, walk around the building 3 or 4 times. The day of the race, we met on the campus of Sacramento State College. This was my first effort to "get moving and enjoy exercising," as I pondered whether "to diet or not to diet."

I know that weight loss is 80% watching one's diet and 20% exercising. So, because I enjoy walking and being around people, focusing on the "20% exercising" was my way of getting started with weight loss. It's very important to enjoy what you're doing, so you can make the most out of it.

## Bringing it Home

My mother had a great shape before menopause. She loved to cook and was very good at it. She would cook the most elaborate dinners for the holidays, as a gift for us kids. I can still smell her food, yum!

As she cooked these meals, she would have several cocktails; her favorite drink was "champ-ale" (a beer, wine cooler). By the time dinner was cooked she was ready to have a good time or a good fight!

However, with the onset of menopause, she started to gain weight. One of the symptoms of menopause is weight gain (and the depression that goes along with it). I saw the effect of this in my mother's life.

My mother was never educated to know that the diabetes she developed later in life had been caused by her diet. Nor did she know that a healthier lifestyle of diet and exercise would restore her health. I think that had her doctor referred her to a nutritionist to educate her on how to cook and eat healthier, she may have had a better quality of life and would not have had to take so much medication.

When I reached menopausal age and began to gain weight, I faced a similar challenge. I did not want to experience the same health issues my mother had.

So when I was diagnosed with high blood pressure and encountered issues with the medication I was prescribed, I started to educate myself about what changes were necessary to live a healthy lifestyle. I found that starting a healthy living plan was somewhat more expensive; however, in the end, it not only lowered by blood pressure but also helped me face menopause.

If I hadn't started making changes in my lifestyle, I would not have been able to bring "this weight" under control. I called it "this weight," because I never wanted to own it. I was determined to remember that it was "only visiting"!

Yet I was not interested in going on a diet. I had never been able to diet, because I found diets too restrictive for me. Just knowing that after I lost weight I would return to the same eating behavior that got me there in the first place, I was sure diets wouldn't work for me.

I had been able to eat and drink what I wanted for years. Now, in my fifties, would I be able to limit what I eat? No way. I felt dieting was too much like having my life controlled. I had to do something I would be able to do for the rest of my life.

I found the resolution when I started to attend college nutrition classes. I learned that it isn't about dieting; it's about health. It's about avoiding heart attack, obesity, diabetes, stroke, IBS, and the list goes on. Now, they had my attention!

So what I am encouraging is not dieting but a new way to eat. Just eating raw foods alone will produce weight loss, because the enzymes in raw foods aid digestion and assist in building healthier cells.

I had to get on board with what to eat and with having more self-control. Yes, I have my moments—especially with chocolate! However, now it's dark chocolate, with anti-oxidants and other benefits. So you can still eat what you like. You just need to find out how to make a healthier version of it. Look for vegan and vegetarian recipes.

I have had to make healthier choices. Even if I am at a barbecue with all the trimmings, I ask myself what foods are there that are beneficial for me. What is good for me? I can still remember when the question I was asking myself was how much I could eat. What was I going to start with? Usually it would be an alcoholic beverage, and then I would pile up as much as possible! Ugh!

I now know how important diet is, and not in the sense of restricting foods or calorie intake. More than that, it is a lifestyle of eating well and filling your cells with nutrients that will help you glow and become vibrant.

Just forget dieting to lose weight; here's the deal: I didn't want to lose my life or live my life being restricted as to what I could and could not do because of health issues. So this was not about losing weight; this was about losing your life! I got it then.

Many women of different cultures do not experience the extreme menopausal symptoms Western women do. Asian women, because of their healthier eating habits, consisting of little, if any, meat and lots of vegetables, have fewer and less severe menopausal symptoms. They call their menopause a "Second Spring," the second part of their womanhood.

Acknowledging what was going on with my hormones and learning to eat healthier has helped me tremendously. I am a happier and healthier woman than I was when I first started the journey of my "Second Spring." I have realized that the extra money put towards my eating healthier is worth it in the long run.

I am worth the effort to work towards a healthy "'Second Spring," because I owe it to myself!


### Knowledge is Power

One example of the trade-off is eating organic foods. We need to maintain the proper quantities of minerals in our bodies and replenish any loss. As the soils in our day are becoming more and more depleted of the minerals necessary for good health, it is recommended that one eat organic foods. Organic goods may be more expensive, but, in the end, they reduce the amount paid for medication.

As more and more manufactured foods are available on the market, local, organic foods have become scarce. Food now comes from all over the country and the world, and you can get into the habit of eating less nutritious foods on a daily basis. A lot of manufactured foods and fast foods also have no labeling, so you don't know what is in it or how many calories you are consuming.

Food is more chemically enhanced than ever before. These chemicals are not natural to the body, and the body may have difficulty utilizing them. Meat is also often enhanced by hormones, high in LDL ("bad fat") and unhealthy due to the conditions under which animals are raised and slaughtered.

Know what you are putting in your mouth! Whatever you put in your mouth goes through your blood stream and is stored in your cells. You want to have healthy cells. With healthy cells you will look and feel good.

When we consume excess food it is stored in the cells as fat, and fat is stored all over the body. I remember looking at the back of my neck and saying, "Ugh! What's that? I have a double neck." I also had fat under my arms. I mean fat was being stored in places on my body where I had never seen fat before. No one likes fat like that.

Don't get me wrong. Fat is needed for the body to be supple and stay youthful looking, that is, "good fat" that comes from natural foods such as avocados, olive oils, and other such foods. What I am talking about eliminating is eating in excess and consuming unhealthy fats, such as fried foods.

When lifestyles are out of control and you are not staying aware of your body, your body can change. We need to make the necessary adjustments as we age, so that we can age gracefully. Disease and devastation can be avoided with proper eating, exercise, rest and lower stress in our lives.

It is also important to be aware of sugar content. Sugar comes in all types of disguises, such as high fructose corn syrup and other derivatives. And it is in alcohol. It is necessary to watch sugar intake and the amount of calories eaten on a daily basis, especially if you eat out, because sugar is in a lot of restaurant sauces and foods. That's what makes it taste so good!

Our diet is important in the journey called menopause, as it helps to alleviate the uncomfortable and embarrassing side-effects. If we are eating the right foods, we will get the proper nourishment and will not need to depend on medications. Remember that our food can be our medicine.

*If you are not comfortable with your weight or you just want to make healthy changes, only small steps are needed.*

Listed below are some examples of what you can do:

*        Choose nutrient-rich foods.

These foods are naturally high in vitamins and minerals and have fewer calories. They are also low in fats and added sugars.


*        Start your day with a good breakfast.

Skipping breakfast may lead to weight gain as you may have a greater tendency to snack throughout the day.

*        Snack wisely.

When you do snack, replace high-calorie snacks with lower-calorie snacks, such as a piece of fruit.

*        Start moving more.

Walk for 30-60 minutes each day.

*        Losing 1-2 lbs a week is a healthy and realistic goal.

Do not be discouraged if the scale says your weight hasn't changed! You may find that you are losing fat and gaining muscle, depending on your exercise routine. This will make your clothes fit better.

### What the Experts Say

Keep in mind that losing a little weight can make a big difference in how you feel by lowering your blood pressure and improving your blood sugar level. Look at the big picture: choose fresh foods like locally grown vegetables, fruit and organic meats (with no hormones: this is not where we want hormone replacement, in our foods!). Choose foods you know to be rich in nutrients where items do not have food labels.

Eating organic helps to replenish minerals in our bodies:

"Do you know that most of us today are suffering from certain dangerous diet deficiencies which cannot be remedied until the depleted soils from which our foods come are brought into proper mineral balance? The alarming fact is that foods—fruits and vegetables and grains—now being raised on millions of acres of land that no longer contain enough of certain needed minerals, are starving us...no matter how much of them we eat!...

"Lacking vitamins, the system can make some use of minerals, but lacking minerals, vitamins are useless...A marked deficiency in any one of the more important minerals actually results in disease...No man of today can eat enough fruits and vegetables to supply his stomach with the mineral salts he requires....Our physical well-being is more directly dependent upon the minerals we take into our systems than upon calories or vitamins." (This information is according to Senate Document No. 264, 1936)

A nutritional diet is essential to healthy weight loss. Also remember that doctors recommend that you get your thyroid checked before attempting to lose weight. Losing weight may be difficult due to thyroid issues. So make checking with your doctor part of your weight loss plan.

And stay active! Regular exercise can benefit you in the following ways:

*        Improves concentration and productivity.

*        Keeps bones healthy.

*        Lowers high blood pressure.

*        Reduces your risk of diseases such as heart disease and diabetes, which are caused by weight gain and/or stress.

*        Increases strength.

*        Helps you lose body fat and keep it off.

*        Reduces stress and enables you to sleep better.

*        Gives you more energy.

The struggle for us to maintain a healthy diet—to eat better and attain a good weight—is a common one. But it can be easier than you think, if you eat well and are physically active. Be realistic by making small changes that can lead to big results.......

## What Do You Think?

1. To diet or not to diet, that is the question: Should you diet? Are you at a healthy weight?

2. Are you often trying the latest diet? Do you worry more about how you look than about your health?

3. Do you feel guilty if you eat your favorite foods?

4. Do you skip breakfast?

5. Are you confused about which foods you should eat?

6. Should you take the time to read labels on foods?

7. Would going organic benefit you and help alleviate symptoms of peri-menopause?

8. Should you avoid meat?

9. Should you add vitamins or minerals to your diet, or should you eat more foods with vitamins or minerals?

10. Does a lack of time or energy keep you from being more active? Why be physically active?

### Further Reading

Dyer, David S. *Cellfood, Vital Cellular Nutrition for the New Millennium: A Compelling Report on a Dietary Supplement that is Offering New Hope for Nutrient-starved Human Beings*. Feedback Books, 2000.

Giblin, Karen and Mache Seibel. *The Ulltimate Guide to Taking Control of Your Health and Beauty during Menopause: Eat to Defeat Menopause*. Cambridge, Massachusetts: De Capo Lifelong Books, 2011.

Grant, Doris and Jean Joice. *Food Combining for Health: Get Fit with Foods that Don't Fight*. Vermont: Healing Arts Press, 1984, 1989.

Kirschmann, John D. and Nutrition Search, Inc. *Nutrition Almanac*. New York, New York: McGraw, 2007.

Mercola, Joseph with Alison Rose Levy. *The No-Grain Diet*. New York, New York: Plume, 2003.

Whitney, Ellie and Sharon Rady Rolfes. *Understanding Nutrition*. Belmont, California: Wadsworth, 2008, 2011.

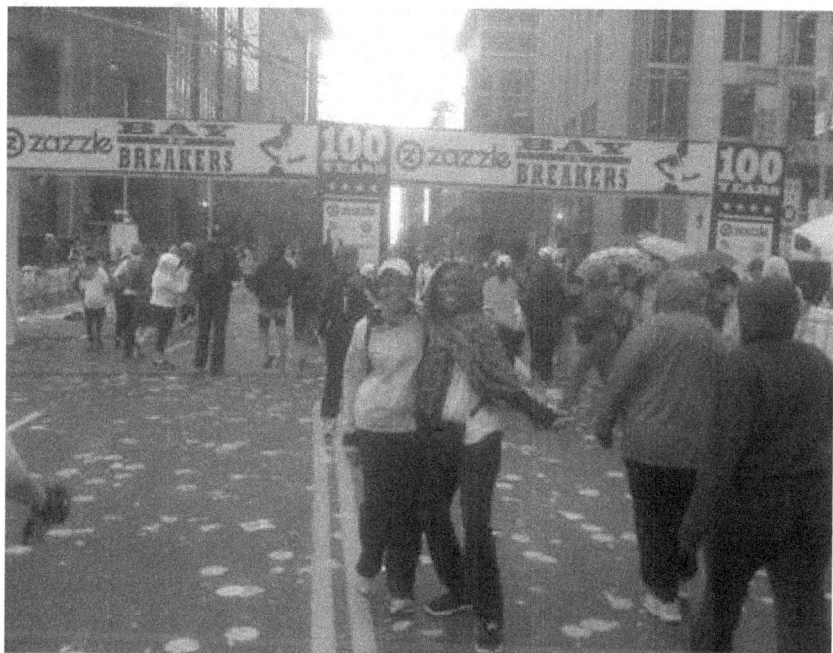

My friend, colleague and client, Sylvia, and I, with our husbands, participated in the Bay to Breakers, in San Francisco, California. We had fun and a ton of exercise! This was a 7 to 8 mile walk and run. A beautiful city......even in the rain!

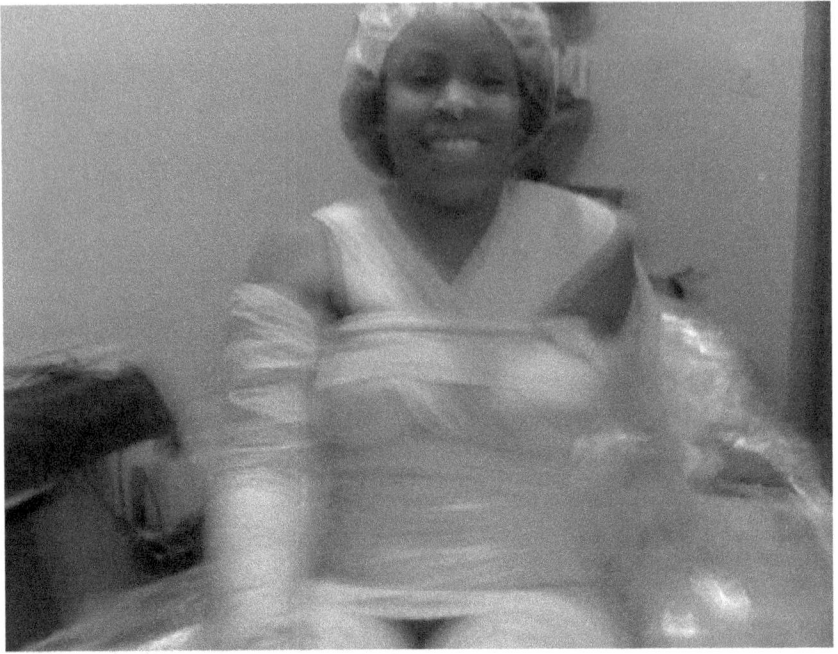

What we women do to lose weight! This is me getting a weight loss wrap on my daughter's wedding day. It worked for the day; at least I felt smaller......if you need to lose inches for the day, this will work.

# Chapter 4 You Know Better, You Do Better

Western women experience peri-menopause worse than women in other cultures. The reason for this may be our diets of fatty and overly processed foods and foods with chemicals and preservatives, etc. Women elsewhere eat fresh foods, mostly raw foods, which help with the nutrient balance in the body. Raw foods also produce enzymes that aid in weight loss.

### From the Stylist's Chair

One day, one of my clients, Sara, began talking to me about alkalizing and how healthy this had made her feel. Sara had always been complaining about feeling bloated. I had noticed at the time that she was looking less puffy and that she was thinner in the face and seemed to be losing weight. She said she had been talking with a co-worker who told her about eating alkaline foods and drinking water. This made her feel less bloated. Sara claimed this really gave her an edge on her dieting program and more energy.

I said to her, "That's funny. A gentleman was just in the salon inviting me to a presentation about alkaline water." And I told him I would attend.

### Bringing it Home

One thing I found that would ease my menopausal symptoms right away was eating an alkaline diet (avoiding acidic foods and drinks, like processed foods and soda). I also learned that an alkaline body is the healthiest state a body can be in.

So I did some research into what an alkaline body is. I learned that by alkalizing your body; that is, regularly drinking 7.5 – 9.5 pH water or eating raw veggies, you will neutralize the acid in your body. I started doing all I could do to be "alkaline," and I started feeling so much better.

Alkalizing my body also helped with my weight management, which was one of the main concerns I had with menopause. I could deal with the hot flashes, night sweats, etc., but weight gain was where you were really messing with my vanity, my sex appeal, my emotions, my everything! Trust me: an alkaline diet worked for me.

When I went to the alkaline water presentation, it opened my eyes as to what leads to a healthier body. This is another step that you can take towards a more balanced lifestyle. It's amazing how different I feel since I started applying these principles to my life.

One thing you should do is to drink five to eight 8-ounce glasses of water a day—this is either distilled water, spring water, or you can buy 9.5 pH balanced water. Although ... drinking this much water is more easily said than done.

I call it "alkalizing." I make sure I carry four bottles of bottled water in my car, and pack it with me for the day. So when I'm in traffic, I just start to "alkaline," just drinking water. By the time I am out of traffic, I have finished two bottles. Then I'm close to having completed my "alkalizing" for the day. You can also purchase alkaline drops to go into your water.

Dehydration can bring on a host of health issues. An acidic body can cause health conditions, such as acid reflux, indigestion, etc. Drinking sufficient water enables one to avoid such difficulties as constipation and dizziness.

Anytime you have a moment, just "alkaline," and before you know it you will have your 64 ounces of water per day, and your body will thank you for it. When you see that your urine is clear, you will know that you are on the right track. We can also get water from foods: fruits, like peaches, and vegetables, mostly greens like celery and cabbage.

### Knowledge is Power

There are three types of enzymes: digestive, metabolic, and food enzymes. As we get older our body loses the metabolic and digestive enzymes, so we have to replace them with food enzymes. That is why we have to eat foods with enzymes that can break down other foods like proteins and carbohydrates (meat and potatoes).

We should eat vegetables in their rawest state in order to digest our food well. When digestive and food enzymes work together in digestion, metabolic enzymes are also preserved.

Also remember our bodies are 70% water. Drinking plenty of water on a daily basis helps lubricate our organs.

Finally, it is advisable not to mix fruit and vegetables in a single meal. The mixing can cause gases in the stomach which results in bloating. Bloating, like hot flashes, is a symptom of menopause. It is not wise to add to the bloating already caused by the menopausal condition.

### *Here are some alkali forming foods:*

**Fruits**
Apples
Bananas
Cantaloupe
Cherries
Currants
Dates
Figs
Grapes-seeded
Limes
Mango
Melons-seeded
Orange
Papayas
Peaches
Pears
Plums
Prunes
Raisins-seeded
Coconuts

**Vegetables** (avoid using the microwave, which kills your food)
- Amaranth greens
- Avocado
- Asparagus
- Bell Peppers
- Chives
- Collards
- Cucumber
- Celery
- Dills
- Garbanzo beans
- Jicama
- Kale
- Lettuce (all, except Iceberg)
- Mushrooms (all, except Shitake)
- Mustard Greens
- Okra
- Olives
- Onions
- Squash
- Spinach
- String beans
- Tomato-cherry
- Turnip greens
- Zucchini

**Grains/Legumes**
- White beans
- Lima beans
- Buckwheat

**Fats/Oils**
- Flax seed oil
- Olive oil

**Nuts/Seeds**
- Sesame
- Almonds

**Sweets**
100% pure agave
100% pure stevia


*Just so you will know, here are some of the acid forming foods:*

**Sweets**
Honey
Doughnuts
Chocolate
Cakes
Cookies
Pies
Molasses
Artificial sweeteners

**Nuts**
Walnuts
Salted nuts
Roasted nuts
Peanuts
Cashews

**Legumes/Grains**
Wheat
White rice
Brown rice

**Fruits**
Canned fruits
Preserved fruits
Artificially dried
Roasted
Jellied fruits
Glazed fruits

## Vegetables
Canned vegetables
Processed vegetables
Canned olives
Pickled vegetables

## Fats
Margarine
Vegetable oil
Sunflower oil
Canola oil
Butter

## Flours
Whole grain bread
White bread
Rye bread
Pasta
Corn meals
Corn (processed)
Cereals

## Dairy Products
Milk
Egg products
Eggs
Cheeses
Butter

## Condiments
Soy sauce
Mustard
Mayonnaise
Ketchup

## Jams

**Last but not least: Beverages!**
   Black tea
   Coffee
   Soda drinks
   Sport drinks
   Processed juices
   Liquor
   Beer
And, of course, wine.

I read the labels on everything I buy. I want to be clear on what I am purchasing, so sometimes I'm in the store for a while. It is important to educate ourselves, to be aware of what is really going on with our food and water supply.

*Here is a tip:*

If there are more than six ingredients in your foods, there are too many. Also, if you cannot pronounce the names of those ingredients, it is not food.....

The foods we eat that are processed or have pesticides or GMOs are dragging us down and killing us slowly. We feel tired and useless. Food is not supposed to make us feel this way; we should feel nourished after a meal, not weak and useless.

It is amazing that food can make us feel that way. We have to take our health into our own hands by being more knowledgeable about the foods we eat. We need to step up to the plate and get our bodies and minds in shape to make the best choices for ourselves and our families. We are all in this together, and I urge all of us to get on board with learning how to eat healthily, in order to live vibrant lives.

Healthy eating promotes good attitudes and good looks, and the view from my window is now clear. Breaking down the word "healthy" says a lot: heal—thy—self! We have the power to heal ourselves.

Now it may seem like this will make life no fun.

Hardly! Because, ladies, this is done in moderation. This is just a list for your information to help guide you in making healthier choices.

## What the Experts Say

According to Hiromi Shinya, Chief of the Surgical Endoscopy Unit at Beth Israel Medical Center and Clinical Professor of Surgery at Albert Einstein College of Medicine:

"Water has many functions inside the human body, but the biggest function is to improve blood flow and promote metabolism. It also activates the intestinal bacterial flora and enzymes while excreting waste and toxins. Dioxins, pollutants, food additives and carcinogens are all flushed out of the body by good water. Water moistens areas of the body where bacteria and viruses can invade most easily, such as the bronchi and gastrointestinal mucosa. The immune system is activated, making those areas difficult to invade. For all of these reasons, people who do not drink enough good water will get sick more easily."

## What Do You Think?

1. Is alkalizing for you?

2. What can you do to ensure that you drink eight 8-ounce glasses of water a day?

3. How can you make sure you're drinking good water?

4. How do you take the time to change your body's pH balance?

5. How will this benefit you?

6. Can you really carefully consider what's going in your mouth and body?

7. How can you make sure you are drinking good pH 9.5 water?

8. How do you take the time to learn and change your body's pH balance?

9. Will you take the time to learn to eat primarily alkalizing foods?

10. Will you buy alkalizing strips to check and see the acidity in your body?

### Further Reading

Crawford, Amanda McQuade. *The Natural Menopause Handbook: Herbs, Nutrition and Other Natural Therapies*. New York, New York: Crown Publishing Group, 2009.

Lieberman, Shari. *Get Off the Menopause Roller Coaster: Natural Solutions for Mood Swings, Hot Flashes, Fatigue, Anxiety, Depression, and Other Symptoms*. New York, New York: Penguin Putnam, 2000.

Shinya, Hiromi. *MNIMH, The Enzyme Factor: How to Live Long and Never be Sick*. Published in Japan by Sunmark Press, 2005.

# Chapter 5 Drinking Empty Calories

In the past, I drank more than I do now. My favorite drink was wine. I thought wine was healthy, until I learned that wine contains a lot of sugar and is nothing but empty calories. My daughter, Nicole, would say to me, "Mom, you're drinking empty calories." However, at that time, I didn't understand what she meant.

### From the Stylist's Chair

Every time I looked around I would get a phone call from Debra, asking me to go to happy hour with her after I finished my day, which was usually after her hair appointment (scheduled at the end of my day). And, of course, I would go, because I thought that there was nothing else to do in Sacramento but to eat and drink. We would usually go to a happy hour where there was music, and, before you knew it, happy hour was over, and there we were three or four drinks later still having happy hour at regular prices! Full of empty calories no doubt!

I had to start declining her offers, because I could not burn those unwanted calories like I used to, and I also could not keep up with that lifestyle any longer. I'm glad I realized this and wasn't afraid to make a change for the better. Debra continues to go to happy hour and is a lot heavier than she used to be, and we are about the same age. She refuses to acknowledge that peri-menopause has hit. She chooses to ignore this stage in her life and not to make the adjustments needed. This is where we differ.

### Bringing It Home

When I started going to college, I learned more about nutrition and how to eat right for my body type: that of a woman going through menopause. I noticed that when I would drink alcohol and eat meats, it would cause me digestive issues. It didn't sit well with me. Before attending nutritional classes, I felt like my life was getting out of control and my body was telling me I had to make a change.

46

I had also begun gaining weight and knew I had to do something about it: exercising, walking, golfing, lifting weights. Then, since I was exercising, I figured I could have a few glasses of wine while I prepared dinner.

I was enjoying this new life: exercising, coming home, popping open a bottle of my favorite Chardonnay and eating dinner. What a life!

Wrong. Little did I know that I was sabotaging myself, because by drinking wine, I was indeed drinking empty calories. There is no nutritional value in wine (except for an occasional, one glass of red wine). My favorite wine was white, with sugar galore: 300-400 calories per glass, and I had big wine glasses!

Sugar, to be sure, is not our friend. We all crave it, but it is the most toxic of ingredients. It is found in most of our foods, sometimes called fructose, dextrose, ose, sobital, or corn syrup, and the list goes on for artificial sugar.

Wherever possible we should use sweeteners that are natural, such as 100% stevia or 100% agave, and as sugars have a host of names and disguises, we need to learn what they are and read labels carefully. It is also best to avoid wines that are high in sugar content.

Not only is wine high in sugar content but it is also acidic and not nutritionally beneficial. It caused me horrible bloating and indigestion. On top of that came my dinner! While the enzymes were breaking down the food content in the wine, here came the rest of my meal, which had to sit there and wait! Wow!

Wine is full of sugar, and sugar is addictive. The more you have the more you want. Fruit and alcohol are like sugar on top of sugar! I was devastated when I learned that fruity cocktails were a cocktail for disaster: too many calories, indigestion, and bloating.

So here's my deal: I decided I didn't like eating anything that was not beneficial for me. I have cut way back on the sugar, and I drink almost no alcohol. I now drink once or twice a month. Since I came to know that alcohol is not beneficial for me, I just don't desire it anymore. Now I am all about the nutrient value of food and drink.

Get to know yourselves, ladies. I observed that when I drank an alcoholic beverage my body temperature rose. That's the last thing you need when you have hot flashes. So I began drinking natural fruit juice, no sugar added. I also mixed fruit and ice and water in a blender for a cool smoothie, and that way I was getting my water intake as well.

Alcohol is something my body didn't need, especially at that time in my life. It only added to my grief. It was one of the reasons why I gained so much weight. With hormone imbalances, a bad diet, and a fondness for wine—oh my goodness!—I had a very acidic lifestyle!

### Knowledge is Power

Let me tell you, ladies, reducing my alcohol intake was not an easy task. Drinking alcohol had become a routine for me. After work: come home, open a bottle of wine, pour a glass, and then start cooking dinner. By the time I finished cooking, I had finished off 2 or 3 glasses of wine.

This felt okay, because I was in my home preparing dinner for the family, so what's wrong with that?

The problem is that it became habit forming. So I had to figure out how to back down from the daily doses of wine. And, to be honest, I prayed about my situation and then meditated on how to remove this drinking wine on a daily basis from my life.

What I did was to remove myself from the environment of the coming-home routine and change it up. I started walking or got involved with other healthful activities, such as working out. So I guess for me it was a matter of replacing the behavior I had become accustomed to with another, healthier behavior.

Avoid alcohol as much as possible; a glass of wine occasionally is fine or your favorite "skinny gal" cocktail. You can make yourself a sassy cocktail with lemon, ginger, mint and sparkling water.

Or, if you're at a social event, you can start with sparkling water with a lemon wedge. You might also order a glass of wine and a glass of sparking water; then, using half of each you can give yourself two drinks to socialize with.

At home, you might try one of these refreshing drink alternatives:

**Cucumber fizz**
1 cucumber sliced thinly
1 16-ounce bottle of carbonated water
1 packet of stevia

**No-calories Vanilla Soda**
1 8-ounce bottle of carbonated water
   3 drops of liquid vanilla stevia

If alcohol is a problem for you, and you feel you are unable to control your drinking, remember that alcoholism is a disease, and, like other diseases, you need to get specialized professional assistance. Just as you would go to an oncologist if you had symptoms of cancer, consult your doctor for recommendations on professional assistance to stop drinking.

You should never feel embarrassed about disease. You may feel guilty, lonely or hopeless, but, believe me, you are not alone. Reach out to health professionals and to others who have encountered this issue.

Whether habit or disease, have courage! You can confront it!

### *What the Experts Say*

The experts say that women should have one glass of wine a day (preferably red); it is good for the blood and contains antioxidants. One ounce of spirits, a cocktail (martini, a skinny favorite drink) with no added sugar (maybe 100% agave or stevia for sweetener), would have a similar benefit.

### What Do You Think?

1. Is alcohol that important to you that you are unable to control your intake or stop?

2. How will you feel once you make the decision to cut back or stop?

3. Does alcohol fill a void in your life?

4. Do you feel that you need alcohol to have fun?

5. Do you need alcohol in order to socialize?

6. How can you socialize without alcohol?

7. If you are around those who are drinking too much, should you change your associations?

8. Do you need to get help with your alcohol intake?

### Further Reading

Hudson, Tori. *Women's Encyclopedia of Natural Medicine: Alternative Therapies and Integrative Medicine for Total Health and Wellness.* New York, New York: McGraw Hill, 2008.

# Chapter 6 Talking with Dr. Tam

My son, Shaun, had originally thought that college was not for him. However, after staying at home for a while with a menopausal mother, he quickly changed his mind! My irritability was always on a slow boil, and I was given to sudden irrational outbursts for no reason at all. It turned out that going to college was, in comparison, much less menacing!

After graduating from college, Shaun pursued a career in basketball. He moved to the Philippines, the country of origin of my husband's mother, and played with a team there. While I was still going through menopause, my husband and I took a trip to the Philippines to visit our son.

### *From the Stylist's Chair*

When I got back from the Philippines, I shared my experiences with all of my clients and co-workers. I brought back some of the herbal tea I discovered and shared it with Nadia, because she wanted to lose some weight before going to Germany. So I gave it to her, and she took it with her to work. I guess she didn't believe me when I warned her to be careful as it works in five hours. It's truly a cleanse.

She took it at work in the morning and by lunch time she was constantly in the bathroom. She said, "I'm glad that my office is right next to the bathroom!"

She was very happy with the results, said she felt like she had lost 10 pounds in one day. She felt that this was not like any other cleanse she had experienced. After the cleanse, she didn't want to eat anything that wasn't healthy nor put anything in her body that didn't benefit her. I'm glad I was able to share this product with her, because it is "a first of its kind."

### Bringing It Home

Back to the Philippines: I noticed that women there are less weight-conscious; they eat what they want. I didn't hear much talk about weight gain or loss. Filipino women seem to focus more on their families, and good food is just a part of that enjoyment. So I decided that while visiting my son, I would leave my menopausal attitude behind.

I soon found myself sitting at a Starbucks, listening to all the Tagalog dialects and watching people enjoying one another. Even not knowing the language, I felt welcomed and at home. I am amazed at Filipino politeness and hard work; that's why, as a whole, Filipinos tend to do well in the States.

I also noticed that there is not a lot of obesity in the Philippines ... in part because of the poverty.

Sitting at Starbucks in the Philippines and watching the women chatting up a storm—women of all different shapes and sizes—it seemed to me that they were very proud of who they were. They didn't seem to have a lot of the hang-ups we have back in the States. It was one of the best experiences of my life to see folks in a culture getting along and enjoying one another. They appeared to love just being together and eating together, friends and family alike.

It was while I was in the Philippines that my son suggested I try drinking the cleansing tea. He took me to a clinic to talk with Dr. Tam. Dr. Tam and his wife own a naturopathic clinic which focuses on natural healing. While my son was singing the praises of Dr. Tam's cleansing tea, I was thinking to myself, "Well, my son is lean. He's not understanding what I am going through." I said to myself, "That's good, son," keep up the good work."

I purchased two shots of tea (100 ml each), just to try it out. I drank it at 1:00am in the morning, as it is supposed to work in 5-8 hours. I'm like, "Right! Here's another gimmick." And I've tried most, if not all, of them!

To my surprise, I awoke at 5:00 am, and the tea completely cleaned me out! I felt like the toxins and the fat were released from every cell of my body. It seemed like my body was thanking me by going back to its natural state. Toxins left unchecked can cause illness and put a lot of stress on the body. You don't want toxins to accumulate in your body if possible.

I took the second shot the next day, and the same thing happened. It's amazing. I lost 2 lbs in one evening, and that 2 lbs was just the waste sitting in my intestine and colon. I thought to myself, "If I would have listened to my son and started this treatment when I first arrived in the Philippines, I might have lost more weight by the time that I left!"

What impressed me most about Dr. Tam is that he has a passion for teaching and healing people. He had previously been a resident of the United States but went back to the Philippines to develop his natural products.

He and his wife changed their lifestyle when she was diagnosed with breast cancer. Now she is cancer free, and the two of them, in their 60s, look great.

Dr. Tam also explained to my husband, Al, and myself what is going on with the food supply in the United States, how we have to start eating whole foods and watching carefully what we eat. We were grateful he took the time to explain what a new lifestyle could mean for us. These days, I haven't quite become a vegan; however, I am certainly eating very little meat.

## Knowledge is Power

Eating naturally, we will spend less time and money going to the doctor for a diagnosis—half the time scared of what is wrong with us. We will know what is wrong, because our bodies will be telling us.

We will still need doctors, but wouldn't it be great if we went to the doctor and he or she prescribed a certain fruit or vegetable to cure what ails us, bypassing the medication and side effects that go along with it. So just be informed when it comes to your health and well-being.

Natural remedies can also be beneficial. Here are some herbal remedies that are considered "natural hormone replacement." These substances are chemically indistinguishable from hormones produced by the human ovary and using them can have similar benefits: evening primrose oil, sage, valerium root, progesterone cream, ginkgo, ginseng, dandelion, black co-hosh, melatonin.* These remedies are not a substitute for a healthy lifestyle (eating well, exercising and getting rest), but they can be good supplements.

***Remember, however, to always check with your doctor before taking herbal supplements, especially if you are on medication. There could be possible interactions.***

Also consider consulting your pharmacist. These professionals are under-utilized by patients and the general public.

**What the Experts Say**

Another aspect of living naturally is to be aware of toxins in your

*** I am indebted to Althea J. Jackson, M.D., for this list of herbal remedies for menopause.**

environment. In addition to being aware of the chemical additives in manufactured foods and the pesticides used in producing food, it is a good idea to be conscious of chemicals in our surroundings. We can't be 100% toxic free, but it's worth the time and effort to find out as much as possible to make our environment less toxic.

According to Dr. David S. Dyer, toxic stress —toxic chemicals and air pollution—are becoming more prevalent in our industrialized cities. Toxic stress is also caused by the increased use of antibiotics. Emotional stress as well has an adverse effect on us, as emotional stress produces adrenaline and adrenal-related hormones, both of which utilize oxygen and reduce our oxygen supply.

Yolanda Williams (www.study.com) observes that life is full of everyday stressors that cause minor irritations. For example, if you use an alarm clock to wake up, the loud noise from your alarm clock is an environmental stressor, as is hot temperatures. Listed below are other common environmental stressors:

* Noise from other causes.
* Crowding.
* Colors.
* Light.
* Insects, etc.

More aggravated stressors include:

* Natural disasters.
* War/ crime and other man-made disasters.

Stress occurs when an event or stimulus requires us to change in some way. Stress is our brain's way of saying, "I know I have to change, but I don't have to like it." Stress involves an imbalance between what's demanded of us and what we are able to cope with or respond to. Stress can build over time if not managed properly, causing several health effects, such as anxiety, headaches, problems sleeping, depression, and high blood pressure. Managing stress is another aid to living a natural, more healthy life.

### What Do You Think?

1. Should you do a cleanse?

2. How would this benefit you?

3. How is this related to your peri-menopause symptoms?

4. How could this benefit you in the long run?

5. Is becoming a vegan or vegetarian an option for you?

6. Will cutting back on meat help you with your menopausal symptoms, such as inflammation, etc.

7. Knowing that most meat has hormones that you don't really need, could you consider eating organic?

8. Can you start by taking baby steps to eating healthier or incorporating nutritional foods slowly to get accustomed to them?

### Further Reading

Giblin, Karen and Mache Seibel. *The Ulltimate Guide to Taking Control of Your Health and Beauty during Menopause: Eat to Defeat Menopause.* Cambridge, Massachusetts: De Capo Lifelong Books, 2011.

Jonekos, Staness with Wendy Klein. *Menopause Makeover.* Ontario, Canada: Harlequin Enterprises, 2009.

Hudson, Tori. *Women's Encyclopedia of Natural Medicine: Alternative Therapies and Integrative Medicine for Total Health and Wellness.* New York, New York: McGraw Hill, 2008.

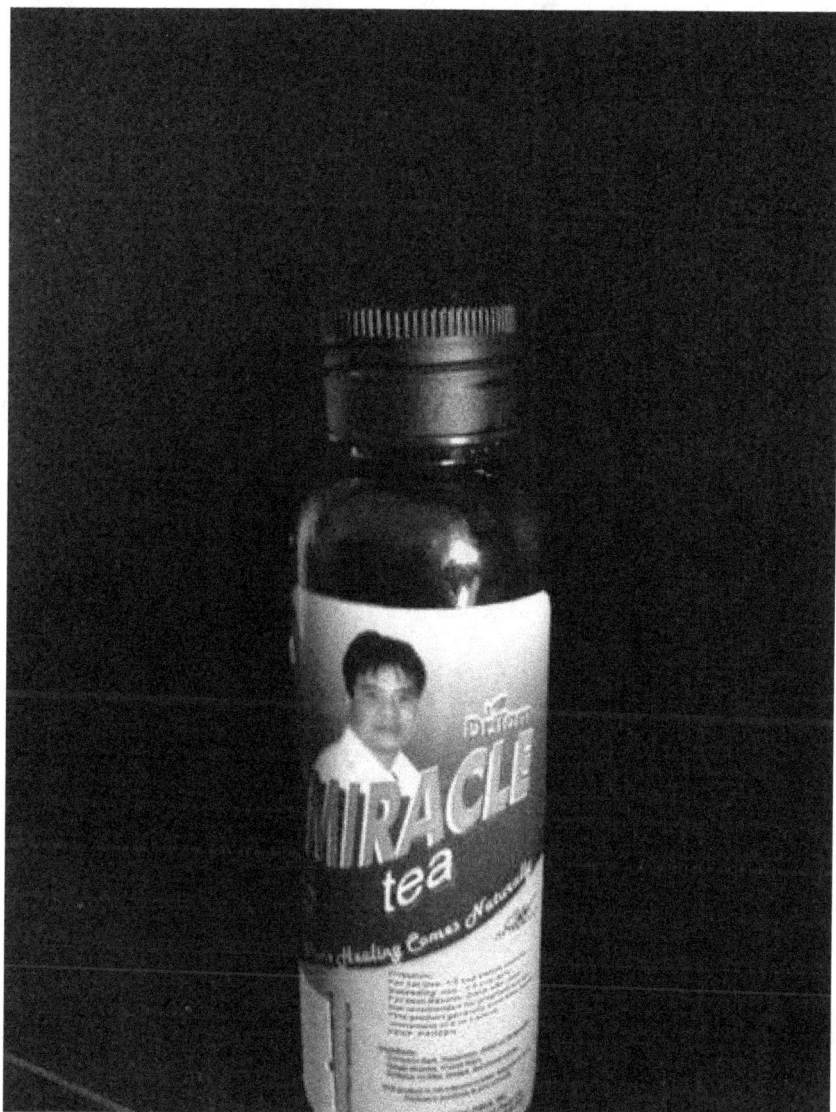

Dr. Tam's small bottle of tea! I drank one of these and the cleanse
began....

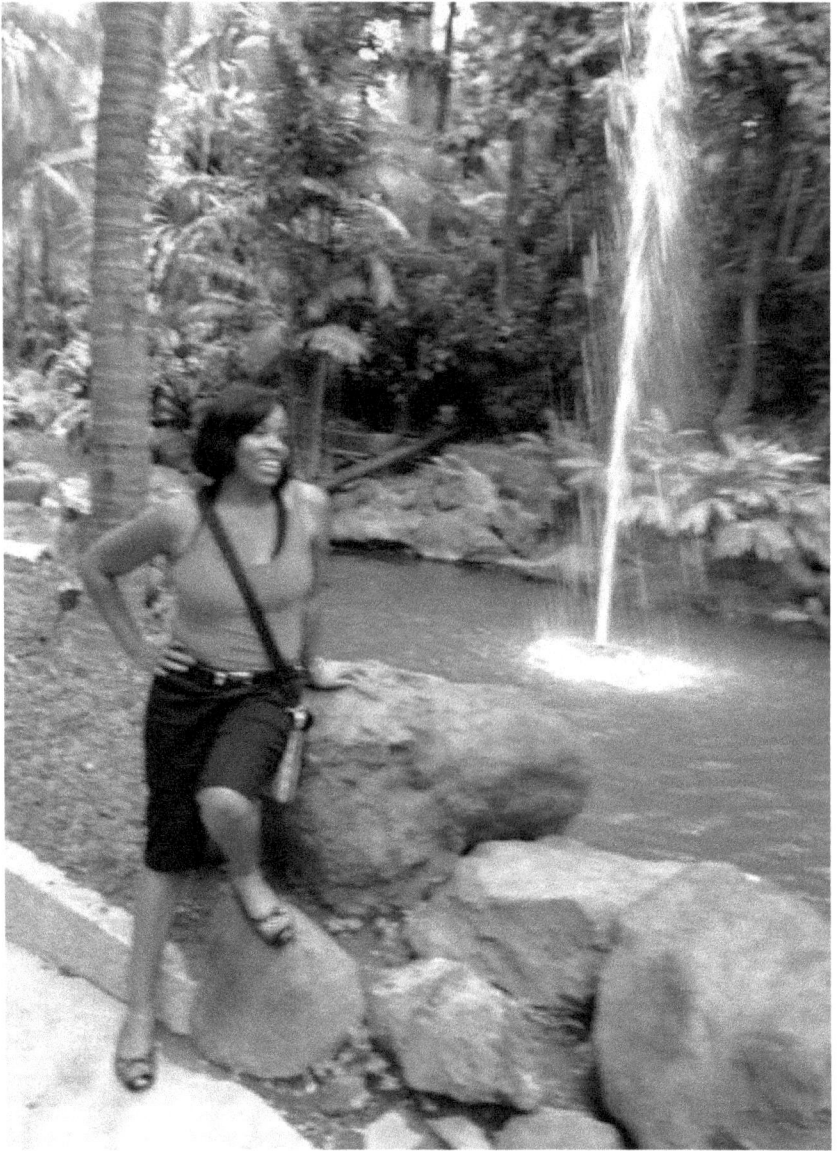

Feeling fresh and clean in the Philippines.

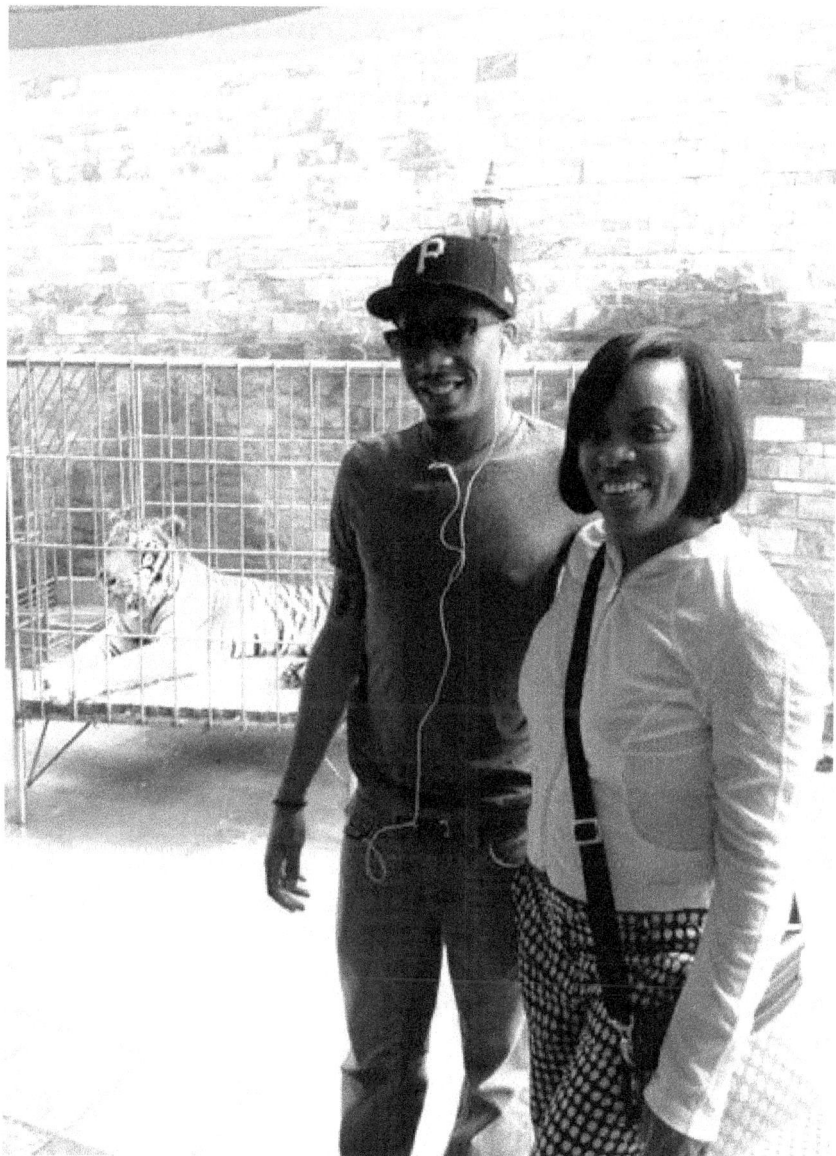

Shaun and I at his friends home in the Philippines. Thanks to menopause, Shaun's was encouraged to venture out as far as he could...LOL!

# Chapter 7 Don't Let No Grass Grow Under Your Feet!

My grandmother, Emma Robinson, was a very sweet person. She worked hard and had a nice home in the Haight-Ashbury district of San Francisco. When I was growing up, I would always want to go over to her house. She kept her home as a retreat—peaceful and tranquil. Every time I went to visit her, her home was free of clutter, full of flourishing plants and bright light shining through the shear curtains in her living room.

I remember feeling the absence of conflict, a peaceful atmosphere of invitation and warmth, like a "big hug." It seemed nothing ever bothered her; she was calm about everything.

My grandmother had a wonderful outlook on life. She used to tell me that she "didn't let no grass grow under her feet." I didn't know what that meant until I got older. I realized that she was always out and about, getting around using San Francisco's transportation systems, which allow one to go all over the city in one day.

As a young adult and now older, I truly understand, because that's how I have been living my life. I am always doing something constructive and useful to enhance my life and my family's life. I have had several employment positions and never went into a job situation saying that I couldn't do something. I have always been determined to do even the impossible, and I will never let not knowing hold me back. I learn and then implement. I'm a good listener and learn fast.

Well, when menopause came around, I started to question myself on many things that I would never have questioned myself on before. I started to doubt my decisions, I was wondering, "What's up with this second guessing myself?" This unsureness was new for me. Once I discovered brain fog and confusion are a part of menopause, I was relieved.

## From the Stylist's Chair

Momma Rosa was her name. She walked into my salon and told me she wanted her hair to look good. She would have a standing appointment every two weeks, because she didn't want to have a worry about her hair.

Momma Rosa was 86 years old at the time. She was always full of joy and positive. I asked her what her secret was. She said she made sure her hair was nicely done and took good care of her feet! She never complained about anything and her mind was as sharp as a tack. She was incredibly smart and would talk for hours about life and how to enjoy it while you can. She also had a strong faith in God.

She dressed impeccably and would tell me stories about her life in Philadelphia. She could wear her fur coats, because the weather was not like in Sacramento, where she had to dress lightly.

I asked Momma Rosa how she was able to stay so positive throughout her life and age so gracefully. She told me that she stayed out of folks business and had a great hobby (... which was crocheting). She said, "Get yourself a hobby and make sure you enjoy it!"

I loved Momma Rosa; she was so encouraging and outgoing. She has since passed away at the age of 93, but I will never forget her or her advice.


## Bringing It Home

When I visited my grandmother, I wasn't going to grandma's house for an array of comfort foods and home-baked goodies. Unlike my mother, she didn't cook gourmet dishes. Food did not hold a great importance for her; it was not a priority.

I have noticed in more recent years we, as a society, have come to use food for more than what it was intended for. We frequently use food to self-medicate or fill a void in our lives.

I remember my grandmother eating small portions and not much. She loved her artichokes with mayonnaise dip. I thought it weird at the time, but now I have come to appreciate artichokes myself. Enjoying and incorporating healthy foods was probably a behavior she was used to in her time growing up.

As a young adult, I never heard my grandmother say anything about menopause, so I wondered if she had gone through it, and, if so, how she went through it.

I believe my grandmother had a fulfilled and well-balanced life, because at age 83, she did not have a wrinkle on her face; her skin was smooth as silk. That could have been how she was able to sail through menopause; she had a peaceful, healthy, "no stress" lifestyle, a lifestyle like a cool glass of lemonade on a hot summer day.

I find myself setting the goal to follow in my grandmother's footsteps. My grandmother taught me a lot about self-love and taking care of yourself. She exercised and had a healthy understanding of self-care whether she realized it or not.

When I began to face the challenge of living menopause in a positive way, I made sure I got plenty of exercise. I did only things I enjoyed doing, walking every chance I got. My favorite was walking through the city of San Francisco, especially across the Golden Gate Bridge. I also started venturing out to other places, such as hiking in Auburn, in the foothills of the Sierras.

I am not a person that enjoys going to the gym; however, I love the outdoors. Since I love the outdoors, I exercise by walking and derive a lot enjoyment while putting in the work. I enjoy myself so much it doesn't even seem like I'm working out!

It is also very important to get a good night's sleep. Sleep contributes to a healthier lifestyle and definitely rejuvenates! It's called "beauty sleep," and we all need it.

In addition to hormone replacement therapy and good diet, I looked to other aspects of a healthy lifestyle: light exercise, the elimination of stress in my life, and finally, a good night's sleep. The healthier lifestyle has aided in reducing my menopausal symptoms. I have also been able to lower my blood pressure. I no longer need to take blood pressure medication.

Thanks, Nana, for teaching me how to engage life joyfully, and peacefully in your own space. Now I am also careful not to let any grass grow under my feet!

### Knowledge is Power

When I was 15 years old, I was a part of the Bay area Big Sisters. My big sister's name was Marge Perkins. Marge was the most amazing big sister ever. She taught me so much, particularly as a young girl growing up in the hood.

She had me involved in many activities; for example, she took me ice skating, enrolled me in art lessons, arranged my first plane trip (to Disneyland), had me doing voice-overs for children, enrolled me in bowling lessons, just to name a few of the activities she set up for me. She put everything she had into making sure that I was well-rounded; I think that had a lot to do with my always wanting to do new things and my not being afraid of failure.

I can remember when Marge was diagnosed with breast cancer. This was around 1976, and breast cancer was not as publically acknowledged as it is today. At that time, it was a dark secret. No one was talking about it, and it was the first time I had heard of it. She would tell me that she was going to be all right and not to worry. On one occasion we had a big sister's party to go to, and, as sick as she was, she got out of bed to take me shopping for a dress. She never complained about her illness; she was always smiling. If she was in pain, she didn't speak of it.

Marge showed great strength and was most gracious throughout her life. She showed me how to be positive and continue to be uplifting for others. She was uplifting for me, even as she knew she was dying. How amazing is that! I will always remember her and her positive attitude. Just writing about her makes my heart swell and tears come to my eyes. We are talking fifty years ago, but she left her legacy with me. She was definitely one in a million. I miss her so much!

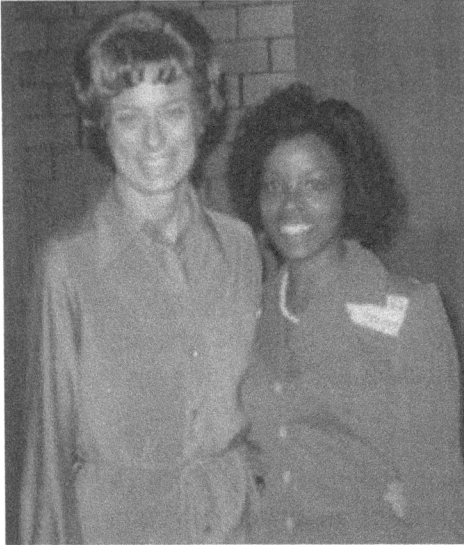

Marge and Marcia at the Bay Area Big Sister party.

### *What the Experts Say*

### *Here are some suggestions that may help you achieve a healthy lifestyle:*

1. Eat healthily—fruits, vegetables, less meat or none, some grains.

2. Drink plenty of water.

3. Take necessary supplements.

4. Avoid alcohol (low to light alcohol consumption, 1 drink daily).

   Please avoid alcohol if you have had an issue with substance abuse or breast cancer in the past.

5. Exercise. Be active.

Make sure you find something that you enjoy doing; power-walks, golf, tennis, or weight training. Involve yourself in activities.

6. Get a restful, good night's sleep.

7. Change your physical space to suit you; make it calm and cool.

Choose your favorite colors, and design the space uniquely for you. This will be your retreat. If you have an extra room in your home, make it your hobby space; create a space where you can be creative.

8. Change your look (hair, wardrobe); make it spicy!

9. Find an outlet for stress.

10. Do not isolate yourself from family, friends or associates. Be active in your local community or faith tradition.


### *What Do You Think?*

1. Do you have a role model for healthy menopause, either someone you know personally or someone you've read about or imagined? What do you see in your mind's eye when you think of them?

2. What does healthy menopause look like?

3. Where are you in your journey? In your "second season"?

4. If you have already passed through menopause in an unwholesome way, what can you do to remediate the negative effects?

5. What would you suggest to women who are about to embark on this journey that would benefit them?

6. What could you take away from this chapter that would help you achieve a healthy lifestyle?

7. Can you challenge yourself to find some type of hobby, exercise, and/or activity that would bring you joy?

8. Are you willing to begin the menopausal journey with some positive behaviors rather than just dealing with it?

### Further Reading

Gittleman, Ann Louise. *Before the Change, Taking Charge of Your Peri-Menopause: Learn How You Can Head-off Depression and Mood Swings, Weight Shifts, Erratic Sleep, Memory Loss, and Other Changes Leading to Menopause Simply, Safely, Naturally*. New York, New York: Harper Collins Publishers, 1998.

Sterling, Evelina Weidman and Angie Best-Boss.*Before Your Time: The Early Menopause Survival Guide*. New York, New York: Fireside Books, 2010.

# Chapter 8 Getting Your Sexy Back

My grandmother was also a fashionable woman and cared a great deal about her looks. She would always ask me how something looked and kept up with the current styles and trends. As she got older, she started to gain weight, but it didn't seem to bother her. It wasn't noticeable weight, because she took good care of herself.

Ladies, I know that the menopausal years are a time in our lives when we lose it, the fashion sense. We develop the attitude, "Well, I'm getting older and going through the change, so why bother?" Nonsense.

It is important to keep our fashion sense about us. This means wearing fashionable clothing, and if you don't know how to go about it, just ask a stylist or inquire at a department or women's clothing store. They will be happy to help you out. Our outer appearance is important, because if we look good in appearance, we will feel better.

### *From the Stylist's Chair*

I had just opened my second salon. I was outside looking at the signage on the window, deciding what exactly I wanted to write (the hours of operation, name and so on). Then all of a sudden I looked in the glass window, and I said, "Who's that?" It was me, and my fat booty!

I was devastated. I had been so involved in building and opening my salon, I didn't take notice of my own self. I had gained so much weight that I thought somebody was following me! LOL.

What to do? I was now buying larger clothes, but I didn't trip too hard because they were still fashionable. This is when I got introduced to Lane Bryant. There is nothing wrong with shopping there, but, for me, I had never had to shop for plus sizes. Now, all of a sudden, this is where I found myself.

### Bringing It Home

Like my grandmother, I, too, have always been into fashion. So, as I gained weight, I didn't let the big size scare me. I didn't wait to lose weight to buy new clothing. Otherwise, I would have been looking dull for a long time. I started gaining weight in 2006, and, seven years later, I was only just getting to a healthy weight.

My view is never mind the weight gain. It's my health that's important. I started to focus on healthy me, instead of how much weight I was gaining and guess what? The weight was not an issue anymore.

As we gain weight we have the tendency to dress down, as if we don't want anyone to see us. Trust me, people will notice! They just don't say anything to you.

It is possible to be a pleasant, loveable woman throughout your menopausal season. When the weight gain starts coming on, just embrace those curves! What I do, for convenience, is to layer up with light cottons or other light materials, so that when I start getting warm, I can then layer down. In that way I am prepared for sudden menopausal sweats.

Remember, ladies, it takes little time to gain it, but it will take a longer time to lose it in such a way as to be able to keep it off. Just stay focused and remember you are getting healthy to lose weight, not losing weight to get healthy.

We should aim to look our best at all times. We don't — literally—want people to see us sweat!

### Knowledge is Power

Always choose clothes that make you feel beautiful, comfortable and give you energy.

* Don't be afraid of color and trying a new look.

Make it a point to go by the fashion magazine racks when you go to the grocery store or the bookstore. Just start browsing through them, so that you can get a sense of style. Browse not necessarily for what is trending but for what colors and patterns go together.

Oh yes, you can also go on the internet to see the latest fashions, just to get your feet wet before you head out on your "fashion journey." You can start adding a little at a time, especially if you're not used to bright colors and patterns. I say start with a scarf; it's amazing what a nice color-patterned scarf can add to your wardrobe.

Ultimately, it is going to take some old-fashioned shopping, actually going to the stores and trying on new colors and styles. My favorites are H&M, Ann Taylor, Loft and Charming Charlies (great deals and a tremendous amount of color to try and jewelry to match). This will be fun, and you can try clothes on with accessories. Make this an event, and take your most honest friend or family member!

* Invest time and effort in your style selections.

When shopping for yourself, make it a special occasion. Spend the whole day and take your time; this way you can browse and make good decisions. Think about if this looks good and is flattering on you, without rushing. Sometimes you will find that one item and it will look great on you; it will be flattering and cover up your imperfections. However, it may not be in your budget. If this is the case, then splurge a little bit. You're worth it, and you will wear that piece of clothing all the time. It won't be something that just hangs in the closet. It can become your staple item (dress, skirt, blouse or pants). Then you can add less expensive clothing for an ensemble built around one expensive item. You'll feel great; get rave reviews; and the process will broaden your fashion sense.

* Shape wear is also a great tool.

As we get older, our body may start going south, and I'm not talking about the airlines, LOL!. So what's a girl to do? Say yes to shape wear! It does help us out where need it. Women have been saying yes to shape wear for over 4000 years, but today there are options for every shape and size. Reclaim your sassy.

* Conceal your imperfections.

Don't be afraid to add concealments to your imperfections. Knowing that while none of us can be perfect, we can still be beautiful. For example, we can apply light foundation with sunscreen protection to moisturize our skin. Moisture both face and body.

* Be open to experimenting with your make-up.

Choose colors that look good on you. It doesn't take much. My must haves are: eyebrows, eyeshadow, eyelashes, and gloss … or a favorite lipstick, keep it simple. Use colors that will punch up your wardrobe (and dress up your wardrobe with accessories as well).

You can make an appointment at a department store like Nordstrom, Macy's, or just walk over to the make-up counter and ask if you can get a make-up makeover. Have an open mind. As they are applying your make-up, they will give you good tips, and, of course, try to sell you everything! Don't be intimidated; just say you'll think about it and buy one or two items. Do not buy a lot at one time. This may be overwhelming if you're not used to wearing make-up. Take it slow.

Try this at home: use powder to fill in your eyebrows if they're thinning, and remember also if you color your hair, take a Q-tip and dip it in your hair color. Put color on your eyebrows and leave on for the length of time you leave on your hair color. Wipe your eyebrows off before you rinse your hair color out.

Eye shadow always adds a punch (usually light on top, underneath the brow, and darker on lid, then blend).

My favorite enhancement is eyelash extensions. This is done if you need them, or if you become a fan of mascara like me. You can put it between your eyelash extensions. First buy some eyelash strips from a beauty store and try putting them on yourself to see if this is something you would like to add to your beauty regiment. If you like them, you then go to a professional and be sure you see their work ahead of time. Know that they do great work before letting them do your service.

I had a bad experience when a practitioner put too much glue on and the eyelashes were too long. I looked like a cartoon character and ended up picking them off one by one. But I do know that there are professionals out there that make them look natural.

* Give yourself a beauty break.

This means you want to remember to relax, refresh and renew. Sometimes we need to take a step back and a long look in the mirror to see exactly what we need. We may just need a spa day, a facial, or some needed rest. Or maybe we just need to make things simple and as natural as possible. A little self-care goes a long way.

* Never compare yourself to others.

When we look at other women, mind you, they may seem to have it all together, but you can be sure every woman has something going on in her life. No matter how good someone looks we are not perfect! One thing you can do to get some perspective is: if you see something nice on someone, compliment them. If you really like the look, take notes. Let's be grateful for who and what we are and keep it moving ...

* Always feel gorgeous.

My mom used to say, "If you don't love yourself, nobody will love you!" Show you love yourself by taking care of yourself; others will see it and love you for that. My mom's saying "Smile at the world, and it will smile back at you" is so true. When I am feeling blue, I just take myself where people are and then begin smiling and talking to folks. That's my cure for the blues. It really works! Because I go out and made someone else's day with a smile; it warms my heart as well.

* Take a beauty breath.....breathe because you're beautiful.

It is important to take time to breathe, to take deep breaths in the nostrils, then release. You should do this ten times a day, if not more. It

71

is calming and relaxing. Especially if you're under immediate stress: just BREATHE.

\* Always look and feel your best.

Even if you are just running to the store or stepping out of the house for a moment, for a walk, bike ride or run, do the essentials: comb your hair, fix your make-up: eyebrows, eyelashes and lip gloss, or balm.

And, by the way, if you're not feeling your best, sunshine really helps!

I can assure you that, in most cases, if you follow these guidelines:

*You'll feel fantastic!*

### What the Experts Say

Let's talk libido!

As we approach peri-menopause, our sexual desire decreases because of hormonal imbalances. For some, having sex can become more like a chore than something to look forward to. If you find yourself preferring to have a frozen yogurt rather than having sex (... my favorite is lemon, yummy!), you may want to express those feelings to your loved one.

Though you may not want to talk about it, trust me, it will be written all over our face!

In the end, sex is a part of life and a factor in living in a balanced way. To be fair to your loved one, your husband or partner, it is good to talk it through, so that, until the desire returns, you can face the challenge together.

Among natural remedies, anise imitates the female hormone estrogen and increases sexual intensity and satisfaction. The Mexican plant damiana is a sexual rejuvenator, aiding vitality by providing oxygen to the genital area.

*Before using an herbal remedy, remember to consult your doctor to make sure it doesn't conflict with any medications you might be taking.*

It is advised that if you have persistent issues in this area, you seek help from a professional therapist. Some men may also benefit from testosterone therapy; consult your healthcare provider if you are interested in pursuing this option.

### What Do You Think?

1. Will you welcome the change and add to your wardrobe as needed?

2. Do you feel the need to enhance your beauty?

3. Will you consult a stylist or do you really need one?

4. How can you benefit from adding color to your wardrobe?

5. How can you enhance your make-up while keeping up with your already hectic lifestyle?

6. Are you willing to work to achieve goals such as changing your lifestyle to a more peaceful and stylish state of mind?

7. Can you be dynamically attractive? What would that be like?

8. Can you bring the romance you once had with your mate back into your life? What steps could you take to acquire a —conservatively sexy, fun, exiting and age appropriate—sex appeal?

## Further Reading

Bender, Stephanie and Treacy Colbert. *End Your Menopause Misery: The 10-Day Self-Care Plan*. San Francisco, California: Conari Press, 2013.

Petro Royal, Beth Ann and Gayle Skowronski. *Sex Herbs: Nature's Sexual Enhancers for Men and Women*. Berkeley, California: Ulysses Press, 1999.

Simon, James and Victoria Houston. *Restore Yourself: A Woman's Guide to Reviving Her Sexual Desire and Passion for Life*. New York, New York: The Berkeley Publishing Group, 2001.

Somers, Suzanne. *I'm Too Young for This! The Natural Hormone Solution to Enjoy Peri-Menopause*. New York, New York: Harmony Books, 2013.

_____, *Ageless: The Naked Truth about bioidentical Hormones with 16 Interviews from Cutting-edge Doctors on How to Slow the Aging Process, for Women and Men*. New York, New York: Crown Publishers, 2006.

# Chapter 9 There's My Wig!

Most women would not connect hair loss with menopause. Yet menopause is the most common cause of thinning hair in women. Since hormones stimulate hair growth, hormonal changes can have a significant impact on the loss of hair. Just as the body goes through a change, your hair will go through a change as well.

### From the Stylist's Chair

As long as I have been doing hair, for over 20 years, I have encountered hair loss. Especially in the year 2009, I started noticing that many women were losing hair. Their hair was getting thin, as though they were balding. Some were experiencing hair loss and thinning hair, while for others the gray hair was coming in fast. I started doing more colors and advising on hair loss.

This was no joke. Women were losing their hair like crazy, and these were women my age and younger.

I remember Ana. When she first came into the salon, she was interested in a weave. As I consulted with her and looked into her hair issues, I saw that she had patches where she was totally bald. I had seen this before; it is called Alopecia, a condition that develops due to stress. I started asking her about her lifestyle, medications she was taking, and stresses in her life.

She began telling me that she had major stress issues. She was peri-menopausal, going through a divorce, raising a teenage son, and, on top of that, her job was highly stressful. To promote hair growth, I advised her to try to eliminate some of the stresses in her life. What had happened in the past was past. If she continued to focus on her circumstances, it would be difficult to resolve her hair issues.

Stress plays a large part in hair loss, but the actual loss of hair will occur about ninety days after the occurrence of a stressful event. So that when your hair begins falling out, you may have forgotten the stressful event that caused the hair loss in the first place. In most cases, however, the loss is temporary.

After consulting with Ana, I installed a full head weave. After a year, her hair started growing back, and she ended up settling on a short style to accommodate her lifestyle. Her life circumstances have now improved, and she looks gorgeous.

### Bringing it Home

I can remember my mom's hair. It was thin, and she always kept it braided, underneath a wig. Her hair was baby fine, and she would have me braid it for her. So I know, for a fact, that the partings were starting to get wider. I always wondered what caused that.

Not only was my mother likely going through peri-menopause at the time, she had other ailments. One condition, for instance, that caused hair thinning was thyroid imbalance. My mother had surgery on her thyroid, and they checked for cancer. Fortunately, it turned out to be benign.

If you have hair loss symptoms, be sure to get your thyroid checked. This may be one of the issues you want to check off your list.

My mother and grandmother were different individuals and encountered their later days in life in different ways. My mother's wit and humor were her way of dealing with tough times. I can remember instances when we would laugh so hard our stomachs would be sore.

Even at my grandmother's funeral, as we stood in front of the casket, my mother looked at my grandmother, laid out so peacefully, and suddenly exclaimed, "There's my wig! I have been looking all over for that wig!" We laughed so hard we cried. People thought our tears were tears of grief, while, in reality, we were laughing at my mother's wit and means of dealing with stress. Stress impacts many areas of our lives.

## Knowledge is Power

Some women, when the stylist is done styling their hair, break out into a sweat. This has happened on several occasions to myself and other stylists in the salon. As a group we have had discussions on what to do in these cases.

The younger stylists couldn't understand why this was going on, and I explained. Sudden hot flashes can overcome a hairstyle, and the client may be so embarrassed about the situation she doesn't know what to do or say.

I would typically just suggest a redo, so the client would feel better about herself. I would always show empathy towards my clients and tell them that it was fine. I understood what they were going through as I had gone through the same myself. That would make them feel better.

As a cosmetologist, I recommend women experiencing hot flashes opt for short, easy-to-manage styles, as well as hair weaves or extensions and wigs. Wigs are now made with human hair and look incredibly natural. If you wear a wig, you will require fewer visits to your stylist and have less embarrassment until the time your sweats are better under control.

Remember, ladies, if you have a weave, even a full weave, or extensions, you must take care of your hair by having your stylist condition and continually clip damaged ends. You should also take your hair augmentations out in a timely fashion.

Once augmentations are installed you should visit your stylist at least once a month to make sure everything is intact. Never leave augmentations in longer than two months; your hair will need to be cleansed thoroughly.

Extensions, wigs and pieces are very popular, as they have always been. These are additional accessories that can enhance your beauty. So never feel embarrassed to wear them. As a fashion and cosmetology consultant, I know that this option is very fashion-forward.

### What the Experts Say

When hair thins or begins to fall out, the hair follicles need estrogen. If your hair is coming out as you comb or brush it, or your hair is unusually brittle or dry, this can be an initial sign your hormones are changing. When hormones are imbalanced, hair will become lifeless.

Hair loss with menopause is caused by the androgen dihyrotestosterone (a general term referring to any male hormone; the major androgen is testosterone). Everyone has some level of the androgen dihyrotestosterone in their bodies. Since the level varies by individual, only some people suffer from hair loss.

The reason for this is unclear, but it is thought that the symptoms of menopause may be an aggravating factor.

### What Do You Think?

1.  How do you feel about your journey with menopause?

2.  What actions have you taken to make this a positive journey?

3.  What physical and mental changes do you feel you have gone through since you began? What would you have done differently with this knowledge and how do you move on?

4.  Am I willing to change my hairstyle after all these years?

5.  Am I ready to go gray and or get a new color?

6.  Should I go for the look that I have always wanted even in my youth?

7.  Should I give up my usual look and go with a sassier, outgoing look?

8.  Can I step out of my comfort zone and be bold and brighter when it comes to my hairstyle? (add hi-lights, cover the gray, it's OK to do this!)

**Further Reading**

Laux, Marcus and Christine Conrad. *Natural Woman, Natural Menopause*. New York, New York: Harper Collins Publishers, 1997.

Redmond, Geoffrey. *The Hormonally Vulnerable Woman*. New York, New York: Harper Collins Publishers, 2009.

Sterling, Evelina Weidman and Angie Best-Boss. *Before Your Time: The Early Menopause Survival Guide*. New York, New York: Fireside Books, 2010.

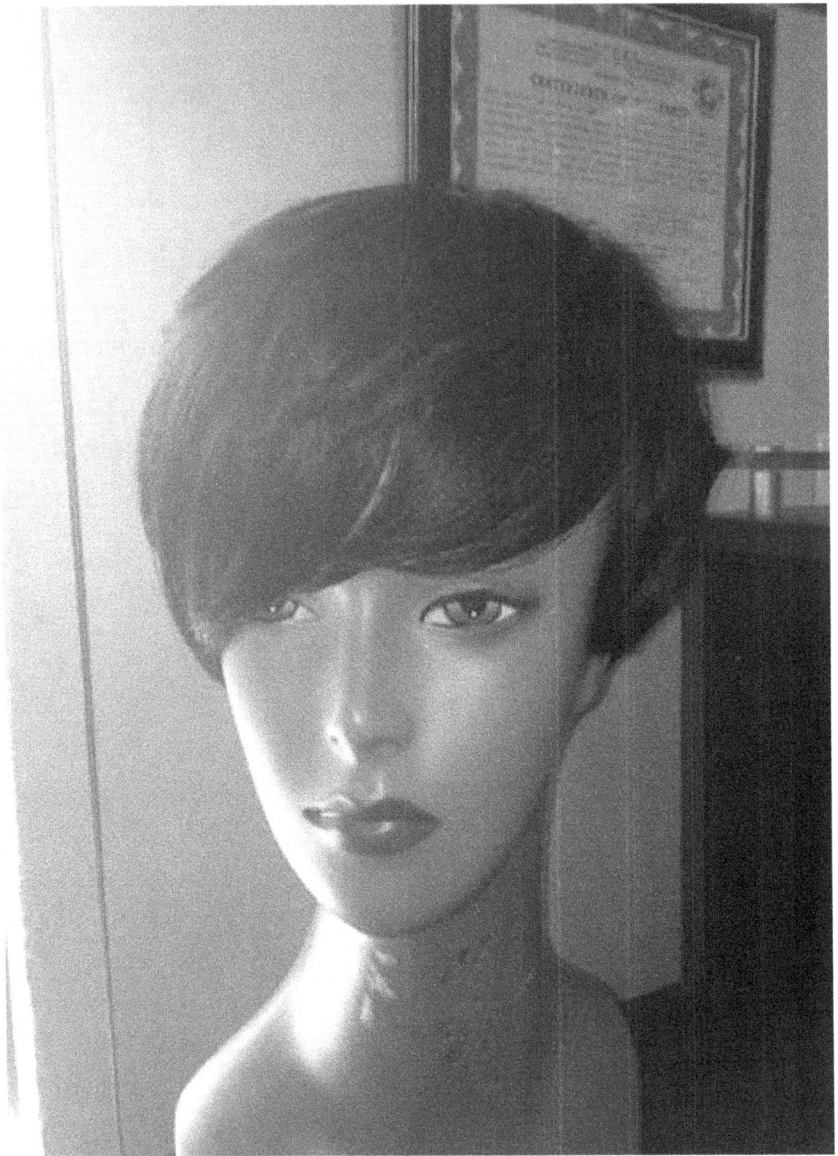

One of my custom-made wigs.....

# Chapter 10  Putting in the Work

Strong healthy relationships and community engagement can facilitate a successful menopausal transition. To remain or become peaceful and joyful, you have to remove toxicity from your life. That doesn't mean that life won't throw you some punches, but at least you will be able to endure it.

Removing toxicity from your life is a challenge; you will have to ask yourself the question: "Do I really want to?" Some thrive on it. So we have to be honest with ourselves and ask: "Is this something I really want? Do I really want to be well, or does it just sound good?"

If you truly want to eliminate toxicity from your life, you have to put space between the toxic ones and yourselves and work on your relationships .... When doing so, you will start to gain peace and a sense of calmness in your life. It may feel strange at first, but then you will have time to concentrate on yourself and how you can become a better person.

## From the Stylist's Chair

Wendy was one on my clients, and her relationship was the most toxic I have ever seen or heard of. She complained that her husband would embarrass her by talking loud and saying to her, or whoever happened to be around, whatever came to mind. He did not have a compass on what was appropriate to say.

For instance, one day I happened to be around him, and he said to me, "I didn't know you were so fat; you sure know how to hide it well." I immediately retorted, "I didn't know you were so blind! (as he had cataracts which made his eyes look opaque and cloudy)" Of course, that was when I was first experiencing menopausal symptoms; I didn't need the insult.

Nowadays, when someone says something stupid or insulting, I just smile and forgive on the spot. I'm a changed woman: slow to speak and fast to listen. I see myself as a student for the rest of my life, always learning but keeping an open mind; never knowing too much; teaching but also listening to new ideas. You can learn something from everyone you come in contact with.

During my encounter with Wendy's husband, Wendy was embarrassed and asked me to forgive her husband. She said he didn't know any better. However, all that was to change. Years later I ran into them ( ... yes, she hung in there with him). They seemed to be doing a lot better as far as communicating, and he wasn't so abrasive — actually a joy to be around. I was waiting for the insult that never came.

Wendy explained to me that she had changed. She had begun to speak up and wasn't going to put up with his outbursts anymore. Wendy became affirmative in what she wanted ... and a toxic relationship was not it! With age and experience, Wendy became less tolerant of his abusive behavior. She was tired of making excuses for her husband, and she became more real and loving with herself. By resolving her toxic relationship with her husband, she became more positive about life and confident in herself.

### Bringing it Home

My grandmother kept folks at a distance, creating a retreat for herself, a reservoir of calm, which others could draw from. My mother, with four kids, three sons and a daughter, was extensively engaged in the community. She had a lot of friends who would look out for us kids while she worked, and vice versa. That was a time when everyone watched out for each other in the community. Whether recounting what happened that day (news flash!) or other events good or bad, it all got around the neighborhood.

My mother always taught me to let my word stand for something and not to say anything I didn't mean. I thought my mother was the best mother in the world. She would help anybody who needed it. She always believed that people in need could have a better life if only they had a little help. She would let people stay with us until they got on their feet, so to speak. My mother was a beautiful human being. She would do almost anything for loved ones or for those in need.

82

I too am putting in the work to build relationships. For me, it was not easy to forgive. When someone would do or say something to hurt my feelings, it was on! I didn't want to have anything to do with that person and just cut them out of life. I would not give her/him a second change.

I can't explain why I was like that. Perhaps it was because I didn't understand what forgiveness was. I would forgive but not forget, which was not forgiving as I would later learn.

Through faith and spiritual guidance, I have learned that forgiveness is not a partial thing; in my faith tradition, it is forgiving completely. In our view, if we want God to forgive us our trespasses, we need to give ourselves completely to forgiveness. This belief and this technique have worked for me in my life.

I have learned not to hold on to anything, because it truly holds me back. My attitude towards others has gotten better, and I feel unrestricted in my daily life. In the past, when I held on to stuff, I could feel my blood constrict in my veins and the tension that it caused me. I not infrequently felt bitter, which was not a good feeling for me. Now, I am able to forgive if I encounter unkindness. I no longer take it to heart.

We women are so important for the others in our lives. We are the communicators. We take care of our families, and they depend on us to lead them in the right direction. We can be examples to those we love by modeling positive behavior, and we can contribute to the well-being of others by being active in our communities.

## Knowledge is Power

In addition to working on myself, working on my marital relationship has helped me tremendously. When I used to get upset with my husband, I would explain every emotion in detail and all that I was going through. I would ask him how he felt when one moment I would suddenly get angry and the next be fine. He responded that he really loved me and that no matter what I was going through, he'd be there for me ( ... while still, on occasion, taking refuge by staying late at the office! ).

For many women, this roller coaster of emotions during peri-menopause is a mess, and we need to explain to our husbands or partners what we really feel at the time we are going through it. We need to have a serious conversation.

Telling and showing our loved ones how much we love them will also help. It can make the difference between a mate's leaving us or our leaving him, due to hormonal imbalance. When you are working on your marital or primary relationship, it is important to be clear and honest about what you are experiencing.

It also sometimes happens that we create a relationship with food, thinking food is safe, when food is what is causing our problems. If food becomes more important than the folks in your life, it's time to check ourselves!

Whether it is diet or personal relationships, you have to be willing to put in the work to make your life free of toxicity and your menopause a joyful journey.

You have the power to heal yourself. You can show those around you how not to be toxic. It's not easy, but it can be done.

*Here are a few suggestions for removing toxicity from your life:*

* Focus on life's precious meanings.

* Learn to smile and to smile more.

* Don't seclude yourself.

* Do volunteer work.

* Tune into your creative side or take up a new skill.

* Dance every chance you get.

* Surround yourself with positive people, family and friends.

* Fall in love with yourself, so that you can love others.

* Learn to give of yourself to others.

* Forgive.

* (... and, most importantly for those of faith) prayer is vital.

I love talking about the subject of the beauty of our bodies and minds and how to maintain a joyful presence while experiencing this "Second Spring" of our lives. Now that I understand most of what I have gone through, I have chosen to be well and happy. I no longer complain about my forgetfulness or my hot flashes, because now I know that this is a rite of passage.

We have the right to speak out about this matter, and share it with others! It is, in fact, our duty to one another.

85

### What the Experts Say

According to Fred Luskin, Director and Co-founder of the Stanford University Forgiveness Project, learning how to forgive can have a positive effect on your mind, body, relationships, community life, and spirit:

"The most important benefit of forgiveness is our assertion that we are not victims of the past.... No one's past has to be a prison sentence. We cannot change the past so we must find a way to resolve painful memories. Forgiveness provides the key to acknowledge the past and move on. When we can forgive we have less to be afraid of....

The second benefit of learning to forgive is how much help we can offer to others. You may not know the power an example of forgiveness can provide. If you look around you will see friends, family, and acquaintances filled with hurt, sadness, and anger. You can help many others with your example of how you overcame adversity and pain....

The third benefit from forgiveness emerges as we give more love and care to the important people in our lives. I know from my own experience and those of many others that hurts from the past often cause us to draw away and mistrust the very people who are trying to love us. Too often the people who suffer from our grievances are not the people who hurt us but those who care for us today."

### *What Do You Think?*

1. How do you feel this experience has affected your family, friends, co-workers, and/ or people that you have come in contact with? What would you tell your daughter about menopause?

2. What holds you back?

3. How do you forgive?

4. How do you fortify yourself in the face of losses —personal, physical and financial?

5. What steps do you take to get to a confident place in life and not feel doubtful?

6. How do you love yourself again, so that you can love others? (not just tell, but show others?)

7. Can you explain to others that you're not perfect and have your faults, admitting that you're wrong and owning up to your mistakes?

8. Can you apologize to people, and love the ones who have offended you in the past, so that you can move on?

### *Further Reading*

Greene, Robert A. and Leah Feldon. *Perfect Balance by Dr. Robert Greene's Breakthrough Program for Finding the Lifelong Hormonal Health you Deserve*. New York, New York: Clarkson Potter, 2005.

Luskin, Fred. *Forgive for Good: A Proven Prescription for Health and Happiness*. New York, New York: Harper Collins Publishers, 2002.

# Chapter 11 Living Well in an Unwell Society

I want, both for myself and for others, a good quality of life, here and now. I feel that life is a gift from God! It is crazy that we so readily look after our material gifts and yet neglect the quality of our lives, our most valuable gift!

Whether you are a person of faith or a person of no-faith, one needs to reach out towards something greater than one's self.

### From the Stylist's Chair

One Saturday, a middle-aged woman walked into the salon, Image Salon, in Elk Grove, California. I greeted her, "Welcome to Image Salon. Can I help you?" She responded, "Yes, do you take walk-ins?" I said, "Yes, and what are your concerns today?" She responded that she needed a relaxer, and I said, "Okay, first I need to do a consult to determine the condition of your hair."

I asked her to have a seat in my stylist's chair. I began the consult and suggested to her that her hair would need to be conditioned before I could do a relaxer and told her I would not be able to do it that day. I told her we could do the relaxer in two weeks, and for that day we could do a protein treatment to strengthen her hair and then a blow-dry and flat iron.

Oh my God! She jumped out of my chair and started yelling. She said she was the client and that I should do what she wanted. She didn't ask for my advice. She started cursing like an unwell person.

I was dumbfounded but not lost for words. I maintained a calm demeanor, because the salon was busy and full of clients.

I just asked her if I could discuss the matter outside, and we went outside. Her husband was parked nearby in a black truck. After she called me and the salon some choice names, still at the top of her lungs, it seemed her husband and her daughter were super embarrassed. She finally got in the truck, and her husband swiftly drove off.

Talk about someone who got up on the wrong side of the bed! Who does that?

A person who is not well in a society that is not well. Whew! I was surprised that I held my cool. But I practiced what I preach, and it worked..... I didn't escalate the situation but forgave on the spot! Apparently that woman was going through it!

### Bringing it Home

As a cosmetologist, I speak with women all the time. Stories of menopause are becoming more and more common, but some women do not have a clue how to deal with it, how to get through it, where they should start, or where they will end up ( ... sometimes post-menopause will hang around for some time). How to cope?

For me, on my personal journey, as a Christian, my self-check is first God: Am I pleasing Him? I know if I am pleasing Him, I am pleasing others, whom God also loves. It is an everyday struggle, but I am doing my best, so that those around me will benefit from the loving-kindness I am taught by God.

We all have sources of inspiration to draw from. For me, knowledge of God is wisdom. As I am wiser in making choices in life, I, and those around me, benefit. God teaches this in *Isaiah 48:17-18*:

[17] This is what Jehovah says, Repurchaser, the Holy One of Israel:
"I, Jehovah, am your God,
The One teaching you to benefit yourself.
[18] If only you would pay attention to my commandments!
Then your peace would become just like a river
And your righteousness like the waves of the sea."*

The closer I get to God the easier life becomes. I learn not just to rely on my own understanding but to pray to God for understanding of my situation.

Knowing God builds character and integrity. Once I started learning about God, I did not fall for just anything; instead I now stand for something. I stand for good morals and its fruits, as in *Galatians 5:22-23*:

> [22] ... the fruitage of the spirit is love, joy, peace, patience, kindness, goodness, faith,

> [23] mildness, self-control.

Each day I choose one of the fruitages to work on. Knowing God and acting on his principles has changed my life. Learning the fruits of my actions and doing my best has made me a better, happier person.

I am also a student of life, continually learning about how to live well in an unwell society. When I learn something new, I am always sharing with those who are not aware but are interested in learning to live a healthier lifestyle. I have a passion for helping others, especially menopausal women.


### Knowledge is Power

The program of the Stress Reduction Clinic at the University of Massachusetts Medical Center uses mindfulness training as a nondenominational approach for people of all faiths and people of no-

* Biblical references in this chapter are to the *New World Translation of the Holy Scriptures* (2013 Revision), http://www.jw.org.

faith wanting to open up to a greater awareness of life. In this approach one learns the practice of paying attention and being in the present, as the foundation for cultivating a calm mind and relaxed body.

The seven attitudinal factors that comprise the approach of the Stress Reduction Clinic are: non-judging, patience, a beginner's mind, trust, non-striving, acceptance, and letting go. Those who participate in the program learn to pull from deep inner resources to heal and begin to cope better with life.

Through mindfulness training one can learn to be more effective under pressure, to live more healthily, and to feel more comfortable with one's self. When we are "at home" with who we are, we are better able to reach out in support of others.

For the person of Christian faith, the daily reading of the Bible can be a source of inspiration. One can find a favorite scripture and meditate on it, making it one's own to remember and use when in need of comfort or guidance. The quotation from Isaiah above speaks particularly to my soul.

Reading and taking guidance from the scriptures has helped me become a better person and put on a new personality:

> [29] Let a rotten word not come out of your mouth, but only what is good for building up as the need may be, to impart what is beneficial to the hearers. *(Ephesians 4:29)*

Also:

> [9] Do not lie to one another. Strip off the old personality with its practices,
>
> [10] and clothe yourselves with the new personality, which through accurate knowledge is being made new according to the image of the One who created it…. (*Colossians 3-9-10*)

Whoever we are, opening ourselves to a greater awareness of life can support a healthy menopause transition. One can start to experience something greater than one's self knowing that we are not alone in the world and that we are all in this together.

It is also healing to accept ourselves with all our faults, shortcomings and imperfections and to realize that our lives are "works in progress." When we fall, we need only shake off the dust, get back up, and try again. Imperfection is simply about trying and trying again until we get it right.

Being honest with ourselves in this way, we are not looking over our shoulders. We have nothing to hide. The effort to become better people, to build relationships, and to work with our communities towards healthy goals may absorb a lifetime, but embracing this challenge can be the key to living successfully.

### What the Experts Say

According to Jon Kabat-Zinn, author of *Full Catastrophe Living: Using the Wisdom of Your Body and Mind to Face Stress, Pain, and Illness*:

"[Participants in the Stress Reduction Clinic at the University of Massachusetts Medical Center] agree to make a major personal commitment to spend some time every day practicing ... "just being." The basic idea is to create an island of being in the sea of constant doing in which our lives are usually immersed, a time in which we allow all the "doing" to stop.

"Learning how to stop all your doing and shift over to a "being" mode, learning how to make time for yourself, how to slow down and nurture calmness and self-acceptance in yourself, learning to observe what your own mind is up to from moment to moment, how to watch your thoughts and how to let go of them without getting so caught up and driven by them, how to make room for new ways of seeing old problems and for perceiving the interconnectedness of things, these are some of the lessons of mindfulness. This kind of learning involves settling into moments of being and cultivating awareness."

Being conscious of our spirituality and meditating on what is real will open us up to who we really are. We will feel the embrace of the Universe or a close connection with God, and we will be able to work with others, each of us in our own way, to make this world a better place.

### *What Do You Think?*

1.  What are you thankful for?

2.  Do you spend time reflecting and writing about your experiences?

3.  Are you connected to a purpose greater than yourself?

4.  What do you want to do with the rest of your life?

5.  Do you want to be a creative, loving, spiritual person or are you holding onto grudges or resentments?

6.  Do you want to be a real be-atch? Are you satisfied with your behavior or can you improve?

7.  Can you endure (put up with) your own and others' personalities and keep it moving with a smile?

8.  The heart grows fonder and stronger with laughter. Can you laugh at yourself when you make a mistake?

### Further Reading

Coleman, Daniel. *Working with Emotional Intelligence*. New York, New York, 1998.

Kabat-Zinn, Jon. *Full Catastrophe Living: Using the Wisdom of Your Body and Mind to Face Stress, Pain, and Illness*. New York, New York: Dell Publishing, 1990.

# Chapter 12 Age Gracefully!

That's how I got here. I am now feeling almost like myself again, like I'm back to normal. It has taken me seven years to get to this place in my life, a place where I now feel comfortable in my own skin. It took a lot of research, attending seminars, and talking with nearly every woman I came in contact with.

As I got deeper into research about menopause —the before, during and after—I tried to figure out what I could do about menopause through natural methods. The experience has been daunting but exciting.

It is a fantastic feeling to know that this journey can be both challenging and exhilarating. At the end of the journey, look what you have to look forward to. To make this a joyful journey is not easy, but if you are willing, you can do it.

We can take responsibility for ourselves and for our own well-being. We can break the cycle; we can take responsibility instead of blaming past generations. It doesn't matter what age we are, we have the right to take good care of ourselves.

We need to become acquainted with our bodies all over again, because this is the present and not the past. This is the situation we are in and not what it was when we were younger. We cannot eat the way we used to nor do the things we did. What is past is past.

We are now living longer, and so we want to live that longer life healthier and with more vitality. We owe it to ourselves and our families to do all we can to assure that the quality of our days is as good as it can be. We are dealing with the here and now, which is: aging in a graceful and loving way.

We can enjoy living a balanced and healthy lifestyle and stepping inside our own, new-found power. We don't need to feel trapped by our circumstances. Knowledge can help us live a better quality of life.

**Here's a menopausal moment:**

I was on my way to Disneyland, one of my favorite retreats. (I like how it brings out the youthfulness in me.) My husband and I were driving through the Grapevine and guess who came calling? Yes, my unwanted guest called "Hot Flash." But now, instead of getting irritable and frustrated, I just rolled down the window and embraced my guest with a cool breeze, and it was a "big hug." It felt so wonderful!

My goal is to achieve a lifestyle that is fulfilling and meaningful, joyful and forward-looking. I feel that life is a precious gift. If I had settled for just "dealing with" menopause, it would have prevented me from living a full and sane life of balance and wellness. I say, "Let us act like the great creation we are. Let us focus on taking care of ourselves and becoming great caregivers of others."

Just take a moment to stop and look at who you really are and what you have in store for your life.

I wish to provide women with healthy solutions for menopause, to provide tools that will enable women to attain a sustainable lifestyle. This means committing to self-care for the rest of my life: eating healthier, seeking information from health professionals, using medications and natural remedies knowledgeably, exercising regularly, participating in wholesome activities, surrounding myself with like-minded folks, committing to a larger purpose ... and, sure (why not?), indulging in the latest fashion!

*It is up to you to take the necessary steps to feel better and look better.*

I am sharing my experience with others in the hope that they too can feel great and look great while going through the "change." Not everyone will be open to the challenge. However, getting better through healing and embracing menopause is worth the effort.

*Let's get well together and embrace our "Second Spring", because:*

# You're Not Crazy! It's Menopause

*Wellness-n-Menopause  Workshops*

*If you are interested in bringing one of these workshops to your women's group, organization, city/ town and or Country please contact me at:*

*marcia_w@comcast.net.*

*These awesome workshops demonstrate how to live a balanced and joyful life. Learn how to live a healthy lifestyle and step inside your own power.*

www.ingramcontent.com/pod-product-compliance
Lightning Source LLC
Chambersburg PA
CBHW070811280326
41934CB00012B/3151